P

From the publishers of the *Tarascon Pocket Pharmacopoeia*®

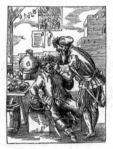

Sergey M. Motov, MD, FAAEM
Assistant Professor Clinical Emergency Medicine
SUNY Downstate Medical Center
Associate Research Director
Department of Emergency Medicine
Maimonides Medical Center
Brooklyn, NY

Rukhsana Hossain, MPH
Maimonides Medical Center
Brooklyn, NY

JONES & BARTLETT
LEARNING

World Headquarters
Jones & Bartlett Learning
5 Wall Street
Burlington, MA 01803
978-443-5000
info@jblearning.com
www.jblearning.com

Jones & Bartlett Learning books and products are available through most bookstores and online booksellers. To contact Jones & Bartlett Learning directly, call 800-832-0034, fax 978-443-8000, or visit our website, www.jblearning.com.

Substantial discounts on bulk quantities of Jones & Bartlett Learning publications are available to corporations, professional associations, and other qualified organizations. For details and specific discount information, contact the special sales department at Jones & Bartlett Learning via the above contact information or send an email to specialsales@jblearning.com.

Production Credits
Director of Product Management: Amanda Martin
Product Manager: Teresa Reilly
Product Assistant: Anna-Maria Forger
Production Manager: Daniel Stone
Marketing Manager: Lindsay White
Manufacturing and Inventory Control Supervisor: Amy Bacus
Composition: S4Carlisle Publishing Services

Cover Design: Kristin E. Parker
Rights & Media Specialist: John Rusk
Cover Image (Title Page, Part Opener, Chapter Opener):
© Wynnter/Getty Images
Printing and Binding: Cenveo
Cover Printing: Cenveo

ISBN: 978-1-284-15761-1

6048

Printed in the United States of America
22 21 20 19 18   10 9 8 7 6 5 4 3 2 1

TABLE OF CONTENTS

PREFACE TO THE TARASCON POCKET PHARMACOPOEIA®

The *Tarascon Pocket Pharmacopoeia*® arranges drugs by clinical class with a comprehensive index in the back. Trade names are italicized and capitalized. Drug doses shown in mg/kg are generally intended for children, while fixed doses represent typical adult recommendations. The availability of generic, over-the-counter, and scored formulations is mentioned. We have set the disease or indication in red for the pharmaceutical agent. It is meant to function as an aid to find information quickly. Codes are as follows:

▶ **METABOLISM & EXCRETION: L** = primarily liver, **K** = primarily kidney, **LK** = both, but liver > kidney, **KL** = both, but kidney > liver.

◉ **RENAL IMPAIRMENT:** Medication requires dose adjustment and/or may be contraindicated with renal impairment.

♀ **SAFETY IN PREGNANCY:** Prior FDA system **A** = Safety established using human studies, **B** = Presumed safe based on animal studies, **C** = Uncertain safety; no human studies and animal studies show an adverse effect, **D** = Unsafe - evidence of risk that may in certain clinical circumstances be justifiable, **X** = Highly unsafe - risk of use outweighs any possible benefit. As of June 2015, the FDA no longer uses letter categories to describe pregnancy risk. New drugs do not have a letter category, and letter categories will be gradually removed from product labeling for older drugs. We have developed the Tarascon Safety in Pregnancy Classification System to describe the safety of drugs in pregnancy. We apply this rating system to new drugs and to older drugs when the prior FDA letter is removed from the product label. Our system assigns the following risk category to each trimester of pregnancy (1st/2nd/3rd):

X: Risk outweighs benefit or contraindicated.

O: Benefit outweighs risk; use in pregnancy as indicated.

?: Risk vs. benefit is unclear; consider alternatives.

For example, the Tarascon pregnancy classification of X/X/X for isotretinoin indicates that use is unsafe in all trimesters of pregnancy. The classification of O/O/X for naproxen indicates that use in the third trimester of pregnancy is unsafe. The trimester risk categories may also be followed by a comment. For example, the pregnancy category for asenapine is: ?/?/?R withdrawal and EPS in neonates exposed in 3rd trimester. "R" denotes that the drug has a pregnancy exposure registry. Prescribers are encouraged to enroll patients in pregnancy exposure registries; contact information is available in product labeling.

▶ **SAFETY IN LACTATION:** + Generally accepted as safe,? Safety unknown or controversial, – Generally regarded as unsafe. Many of our "+" listings are from the AAP policy "The Transfer of Drugs and Other Chemicals Into Human Milk" (see www.aap.org) and may differ from those recommended by the manufacturer.

© **DEA CONTROLLED SUBSTANCES: I** = High abuse potential, no accepted use (e.g., heroin, marijuana), **II** = High abuse potential and severe dependence liability (e.g., morphine, codeine, hydromorphone, cocaine, amphetamines, methylphenidate, secobarbital). Some states require triplicates. **III** = Moderate dependence liability (e.g., *Tylenol #3*, *Vicodin*), **IV** = Limited dependence liability (benzodiazepines, propoxyphene, phentermine), **V** = Limited abuse potential (e.g., *Lomotil*).

$ RELATIVE COST: Cost codes used are "per month" of maintenance therapy (e.g., antihypertensives) or "per course" of short-term therapy (e.g., antibiotics). Codes are calculated using average wholesale prices (at press time in US dollars) for the most common indication and route

Code	Cost
$	< $25
$$	$25 to $49
$$$	$50 to $99
$$$$	$100 to $199
$$$$$	≥ $200

of each drug at a typical adult dosage. For maintenance therapy, costs are calculated based upon a 30-day supply or the quantity that might typically be used in a given month. For short-term therapy (i.e., 10 days or less), costs are calculated on a single treatment course. When multiple forms are available (e.g., generics), these codes reflect the least expensive generally available product. When drugs don't neatly fit into the classification scheme above, we have assigned codes based upon the relative cost of other similar drugs. *These codes should be used as a rough guide only*, as (1) they reflect cost, not charges, (2) pricing often varies substantially from location to location and time to time, and (3) HMOs, Medicaid, and buying groups often negotiate quite different pricing. Check with your local pharmacy if you have any questions.

▪ BLACK BOX WARNINGS: This icon indicates that there is a black box warning associated with this drug. Note that the warning itself is not listed.

FOREWORD

Is pain the fifth vital sign? It may be, but what is the normal range? The movement to be certain that every patient was pain-free by prescribing an opioid is clearly now seen as misguided. Relief of pain, as a manifestation of disease and a disease entity unto itself, is certainly a central tenet of good medicine. However, pain management implies just that - that the physician and patient work together to make the pain manageable. That requires the physician to be extraordinarily skilled with all sorts of approaches to the treatment of pain — bringing relief and avoiding harm in the short and long term.

There is no doubt that had this book been written 20 years ago it would have had a rather small audience. Now, because of voices like the author's, we acknowledge the depth and breadth of the information collected here as essential to the practice of Emergency Medicine. This book couples the enlightened, evidence-based principles and approach created by the author with the peer-reviewed power of the *Tarascon Pharmacopeia*. It will be a reference for much of my practice and teaching, as it should yours.

Richard J. Hamilton, MD
Editor-In-Chief Tarascon *Pocket Pharmacopoeia*
Professor and Chief, Department of Emergency Medicine
Drexel University College of Medicine
Philadelphia, PA

OPIOID EQUIVALENCY*

Opioid	PO	IV/SC/IM
buprenorphine	n/a	0.3–0.4 mg
butorphanol	n/a	2 mg
codeine	130 mg	75 mg
fentanyl	?	0.1 mg
hydrocodone	20 mg	n/a
hydromorphone	7.5 mg	1.5 mg
levorphanol	4 mg	2 mg
meperidine	300 mg	75 mg
methadone	5–15 mg	2.5–10 mg
morphine	30 mg	10 mg
nalbuphine	n/a	10 mg
oxycodone	20 mg	n/a
oxymorphone	10 mg	1 mg
pentazocine	50 mg	30 mg

*Approximate equianalgesic doses as adapted from the 2003 American Pain Society (www.ampainsoc.org) guidelines and the 1992 AHCPR guidelines. n/a = Not available. See drug entries themselves for starting doses. Many recommend initially using lower than equivalent doses when switching between different opioids. IV doses should be titrated slowly with appropriate monitoring. All PO dosing is with immediate-release preparations. Individualize all dosing, especially in the elderly, children, and in those with chronic pain, opioid naïve, or hepatic/renal insufficiency.

PRINCIPLES OF SAFE AND EFFECTIVE EMERGENCY DEPARTMENT (ED) PAIN MANAGEMENT

A provision of timely, effective, and safe analgesia is a specialty-defining skill of emergency department (ED) clinicians. In light of the current opioid crisis affecting the lives of millions of people across the nation, ED clinicians have a unique opportunity to combat this epidemic by judicious and safe opioid prescribing in the ED and at discharge and actively participating in identifying, referring, and even initiating treatment for patients with opioid use disorder. This opportunity is based on several key principles that were published by the American Academy of Emergency Medicine and American College of Emergency Physicians in 2017 as well as 2016 CDC Guidelines for Prescribing Opioids for Chronic Pain. Below is a summary of these recommendations.

General Principles of Acute Pain Management

1. Management of acute pain in the ED should be patient-centered and pain syndrome-specific by utilizing a multimodal approach that includes non-pharmacological and pharmacological modalities of non-opioid and opioid analgesics.
2. Assessment of acute pain should be based on a need for analgesia to improve and/or restore patients' functional status when feasible, rather than patient-reported pain scores.
3. ED clinicians should engage patients in shared decision-making about overall treatment goals, expectations, and the natural trajectory of the specific painful condition, as well as analgesic options including short- and long-term

1

benefits and risks of adverse effects associated with their use.

4. When opioids are used for acute pain, ED clinicians should make every effort to combine them with non-pharmacologic and non-opioid pharmacological therapies (i.e., yoga, exercise, cognitive behavioral therapy, complementary/alternative medical therapies), NSAIDs, acetaminophen, topical analgesics, and nerve blocks, etc.

5. When considering opioids for acute pain, ED clinicians should involve patients in shared decision-making about analgesic options, opioid alternatives, risks and benefits of opioid therapies, expectations about the pain trajectory, and management approaches.

6. When considering opioids for acute pain, ED clinicians should counsel patients regarding serious adverse effects such as sedation, respiratory depression, pruritus, constipation, rapid development of tolerance, hyperalgesia, dependence, addiction, overdose, and death.

7. Should the duration of acute pain extend beyond the expected course, complications of acute painful syndrome should be ruled out, and a trial of non-opioid therapy and non-pharmacological therapy should be considered.

8. When considering administration of opioids for acute pain, ED clinicians should consider accessing the respective state's Prescription Drug Monitoring Program (PDMP). The data retrieved from PDMPs can be used to identify excessive dosages and dangerous combinations as well as patients with suspected/diagnosed opioid use disorder in order to offer counseling and referral for addiction treatment.

Pharmacological Options

▶ *Non-Opioid Analgesics*

1. Non-steroidal anti-inflammatory drugs (NSAIDs) should be administered at their lowest effective analgesic dose (analgesic ceiling dose), both in the ED and upon discharge, for the shortest treatment course.

2. There is no appreciable difference with respect to analgesic efficacy between NSAIDs (ibuprofen, naproxen, ketorolac, diclofenac) commonly used in the ED.

3. Oral and/or parenteral NSAIDs should be used with great caution (or not at all) in elderly patients and/or patients at risk for or with established renal insufficiency, heart failure, or gastrointestinal hemorrhage.

4. When a patient's acutely painful condition (e.g., sprains, strains, bruises, small fractures) is deemed appropriate for treatment with an NSAID, but there are contraindications to their systemic use, strong consideration should be given to topical preparations (e.g., diclofenac gel or patches).

5. Oral and rectal forms of acetaminophen, either alone or in combination with other analgesics, provide similar analgesia to intravenous acetaminophen but with slower onset of action. For patients who have contraindications to oral and rectal routes and warrant acetaminophen, the intravenous route might be considered.

6. Regional (ultrasound-guided) and local nerve blocks should be strongly considered for traumatic and nontraumatic painful conditions, either alone or in combination with pharmacological and non-pharmacological treatment modalities in the ED.

7. Subdissociative dose ketamine (SDK), administered either as an adjunct to opioid and non-opioid analgesics or as a single agent, may be considered in the ED for managing a variety of acute and chronic painful conditions. ED patients should be counseled about the potential for minor but bothersome psychoperceptual side effects, which occur at a relatively high rate.

8. Limited evidence supports the use of intravenous lidocaine for several specific painful conditions in the ED (renal colic, herpetic/post-herpetic neuralgia); it might be considered for patients without preexisting structural heart disease and rhythm disturbances.

9. Trigger-point injections with local anesthetics (lidocaine, bupivacaine) might be considered for patients with acute myofascial painful syndromes.

10. Nitrous oxide should be considered for the treatment of acute painful conditions (predominantly traumatic) in the ED, either alone or as an adjunct to other analgesic modalities.

▶ *Opioid Analgesics*

1. When feasible, emergency medicine (EM) clinicians should make every effort to utilize non-pharmacological modalities and non-opioid analgesics to alleviate pain in the ED and especially on discharge. They are encouraged to use opioid analgesics only when the benefits of opioids are believed to outweigh the risks (not routinely).

2. **Parenteral opioids** are effective, inexpensive, and rapidly reversible analgesics that quickly relieve acute pain in the ED.

3. Parenteral opioids must be titrated regardless of their initial dosing regimens (weight-based or fixed) until pain is optimized to acceptable level (functionality status) or side effects become intolerable.

4. Patients should be engaged in shared-decision making regarding the type, dose, and route of parenteral opioid administration, as repetitive attempts of IV cannulation and intramuscular injections are associated with pain. In addition, intramuscular injections are associated with unpredictable absorption rates and complications such as muscle necrosis, muscle fibrosis, soft tissue infection, and the need for dose escalation.

5. Morphine sulfate provides better balance of analgesic efficacy and safety among all parenteral opioids due to lesser degree of lipophilicity.

6. Hydromorphone should be avoided as a first-line opioid analgesic in the ED due to significant euphoria and severe respiratory depression requiring naloxone reversal predominantly related to higher lipophilicity. Its use should be reserved for patients with painful syndromes that are intractable or multi-analgesic-resistant.

7. Extreme caution should be executed when parenteral opioids are administered to patients with renal insufficiency and/or renal failure by utilizing lower initial doses and extending the dosing intervals.

8. When intravascular access is unobtainable, EM clinicians should consider utilization of intranasal (fentanyl), nebulized (fentanyl and morphine), or transmucosal (rapidly dissolvable fentanyl tablets) routes of analgesic administration for patients with acute painful conditions.

9. Oral opioids are effective for managing a variety of acute painful conditions of moderate to severe intensity in the ED; however, there is no appreciable analgesic difference between commonly used opioids (e.g., oxycodone, hydrocodone, and morphine sulfate immediate release [MSIR]).

10. When oral opioids are used for acute pain, the lowest effective dose and fewest number of tablets needed should be prescribed. In most cases, less than 3 days' worth of medication is necessary, and rarely is more than 5 days' worth needed.

11. If the painful condition outlasts a 3-day supply, re-evaluation in a healthcare facility is beneficial.

12. EM clinicians should only prescribe immediate-release (short-acting) formulary in the ED and at discharge.

13. EM clinicians should not prescribe long-acting, extended-release, or sustained-release opioid formulations, which include both oral and transdermal (fentanyl) medications in the ED. These formulations are not indicated for acute pain and carry a high risk of overdose, particularly in opioid-naïve patients.

14. ED providers should counsel patients about safe medication storage and disposal, as well as the consequences of a failure to do so; potential for abuse and misuse by others (teens and young adults) and potential for overdose and death (children and teens).

Non-Pharmacological Management

1. ED clinicians should consider applications of heat or cold and specific recommendations for activity and exercise, and/or early referral to physical therapy.

2. The use of alternative and complementary therapies, such as acupuncture, guided imagery, cognitive behavioral therapy, and hypnosis, has not been systematically evaluated for use in the ED. In general, their application may be limited in the context of an ED, although continued investigation into their safety and efficacy is strongly encouraged.

3. ED clinicians might consider utilization of osteopathic manipulation techniques (high-velocity, low-amplitude techniques, muscle energy techniques, and soft tissue techniques) for patients presenting to the ED with pain syndromes of skeletal, arthrodial, and myofascial origins.

General Principles of Chronic Non-Cancer Pain (CNCP) Management

1. Management of chronic non-cancer pain (exacerbation) in the ED should be patient-centered and pain syndrome-specific by utilizing a multimodal approach that primarily includes non-pharmacological and non-opioid analgesic modalities.

2. Opioid analgesics should not be routinely prescribed in the ED for patients with CNCP and should only be considered on a case-by-case basis when benefits for alleviating pain and improving functionality outweigh the risks of short-term and long-term adverse effects.

3. ED clinicians should engage patients in shared decision-making about overall treatment goals and expectations, the natural trajectory of patients' specific painful condition, and analgesic options, including short-term and long-term benefits as well as the risks of adverse effects associated with their use.

4. ED clinicians should counsel patients with CNCP that care for their painful conditions should be coordinated and managed by a single provider with expertise in this disease.

5. When considering opioids for CNCP, ED clinicians should involve patients in shared decision-making about analgesic options, opioid alternatives, the risks and benefits of opioid therapies, rational expectations about the pain trajectory, and management approach.

6. When considering opioids for CNCP, ED clinicians should counsel patients regarding serious adverse effects associated with their use, such as sedation, respiratory depression, pruritus, constipation, rapid development of tolerance, hyperalgesia, dependence, addiction, overdose, and death.

7. When opioids are used at discharge for patients with CNCP, the lowest effective dose and fewest number of tablets needed should be prescribed. In most cases, less than 3 days' worth is necessary and rarely is more than 5 days' worth needed.

8. EM clinicians should not prescribe long-acting, extended-release, or sustained-release opioid formulations, which include both oral and transdermal (fentanyl) medications in the ED and at discharge for managing CNCP.

9. EM clinicians should avoid prescribing opioids to patients with CNCP who are taking sedative-hypnotics (benzodiazepines), as these drug-drug interactions can lead to higher rates of morbidity and mortality.

References

1. Motov S, Strayer R, Hayes B, et al. AAEM White Paper on Acute Pain Management in the Emergency Department. Available at www

.aaem.org/UserFiles/file/WhitePaperAcutePainManaginED102417
.pdf (posted October 24, 2017; accessed February 22, 2018).

2. Optimizing the Treatment of Acute Pain Management in the Emergency Department. *Ann Emerg Med.* 2017;70(3):446–448.

3. Centers for Disease Control and Prevention. CDC Guideline for Prescribing Opioids for Chronic Pain. Available at www.cdc.gov /drugoverdose/prescribing/guideline.html (updated August 29, 2017; accessed on February 22, 2018).

THE CERTA CONCEPT

The CERTA (channels/enzymes/receptors targeted analgesia) concept is based on our improved understanding of the neuro-biological aspects of pain, with a shift from a symptom-based approach to a mechanistic approach. This patient-specific, pain syndrome-targeted analgesic approach is geared toward a broader utilization of non-opioid analgesics with a more refined and judicious use of opioids. These synergistic combinations of different classes of analgesics acting on different target sites will result in greater analgesia, reduced dose of each individual medication (potentially leading to fewer side effects), greater patient satisfaction, shorter length of stay in the ED, and better overall ED throughput. In addition, this concept will allow us to administer non-opioid analgesics as the first-line therapeutics for managing a variety of acute and chronic painful syndromes in the ED and utilize opioids as rescue analgesics. The ultimate goal of CERTA is to equip ED clinicians with a variety of pharmacological and non-pharmacological (yoga, acupuncture, iontophoresis, physical therapy, and cognitive-behavioral therapy) therapeutic modalities to provide patient-specific, pain syndrome-targeted analgesia. An example of this concept would include a combination of a COX enzyme inhibitor (ketorolac) with a sodium channel blocking agent (IV lidocaine) for patients with renal colic. Another example would include a combination of NMDA-receptor antagonist (ketamine) with sodium channel blockade (lidocaine via ultrasound-guided nerve blocks) for acute traumatic musculoskeletal pain; combination of a COX enzyme inhibitor (ibuprofen) with calcium channel blocking agents (either gabapentin or pregabalin) and sodium channel

11

blocking agent (lidocaine patch) for neuropathic pain; and combination of antidopaminergic agents (metoclopramide, prochlorperazine) with a COX enzyme inhibitor (ketorolac) and/or sodium channel blockade (lidocaine/bupivacaine for paracervical blocks) for patients with tension or migraine-type headache.

The table below summarizes different classes of analgesics targeting channels, enzymes, or receptors in order to manage pain in the ED.

Sodium Channel Blocking Agents (Target Site)	
Medications	**Pain Syndromes**
Local Anesthetics: **Articane:** 4% **Bupivacaine** w/o epi: 0.25–0.5% **Bupivacaine** with epi: 0.25–0.5% **Chloroprocaine** 2–3% **Lidocaine** w/o epi: 0.5–2% **Lidocaine** with epi: 0.5–2% **Mepivacaine:** 1–2% **Prilocaine:** 4% **Procaine:** 0.25–0.5% **Ropivacaine:** 0.2 –1% **Tetracaine:** 0.5% eye drops	Acute Musculoskeletal Pain (fractures, dislocations, subluxations, muscle sprains, strains, spasms) Acute Soft Tissue Pain (laceration, abscess, foreign bodies) Acute Visceral Pain (renal colic) Acute Neuropathic Pain (acute herpetic neuralgia) Acute Corneal Abrasion (tetracaine) Chronic Musculoskeletal Pain (flare of rheumatoid arthritis, osteoarthritis) Chronic Neuropathic Pain (postherpetic neuralgia, trigeminal neuralgia)

(*continues*)

Antidepressants: Nortriptyline, Amitriptyline	Chronic Neuropathic Pain (post-herpetic neuralgia, trigeminal neuralgia)

Calcium Channel (central) Blocking Agents (Target Site)	
Medications	**Pain Syndromes**
Gabapentin, Pregabalin	Acute Post-Operative Pain
	Acute Neuropathic Pain
	Chronic Neuropathic Pain (nerve palsies, neuralgias, diabetic neuropathy, post-herpetic neuropathy, sciatica, fibromyalgia)

COX-1, COX-2 Enzyme Inhibitors (Target Site)	
Medications	**Pain Syndromes**
NSAIDs: Ibuprofen Naproxen Diclofenac Ketoprofen Ketorolac	Acute Musculoskeletal Pain (sprains, strains, contusions, fractures, dislocations, subluxations, tendinopathies, arthralgias, back pain)
	Acute Visceral Pain (renal and biliary colic, abdominal pain)
	Acute Soft Tissue Pain (lacerations, contusions, foreign bodies, abscesses)
	Acute Headache
Acetaminophen (additional possible COX-3 inhibition)	Chronic Musculoskeletal Pain (osteoarthritis, rheumatoid arthritis, gout)

(continues)

Central Alpha 1, 2 Receptor Agonist (Target Site)	
Medications	**Pain Syndromes**
Clonidine	Acute Pain
Dexmedetomidine	Chronic Pain (neuropathic pain, vaso-occlusive sickle cell painful crisis)

D1-2 Receptor Antagonists (Target Site)	
Medications	**Pain Syndromes**
Haloperidol	Acute Pain (migraine headache)
Droperidol	Chronic Abdominal Pain
Metoclopramide	Cyclic Vomiting Syndrome
Prochlorperazine	Gastroparesis
Chlorpromazine	

GABA Receptor Agonist/NMDA Antagonist (Target Site)	
Medications	**Pain Syndromes**
Propofol	Intractable Migraine Headache

5HT-2, 5HT-3 Receptor Antagonists (Target Site)	
Medications	**Pain Syndromes**
Metoclopramide	Acute Pain (migraine headache)
Haldol	Chronic Abdominal Pain
Droperidol	Cyclic Vomiting Syndrome

(*continues*)

5HT-1 Receptor Agonists (Target Site)	
Medications	**Pain Syndromes**
Sumatriptan	Acute Pain (migraine headache, cluster headache)

NMDA/Glutamate Receptor Antagonists (Target Site)	
Medications	**Pain Syndromes**
Ketamine Magnesium	**Acute Traumatic/Non-Traumatic Pain:** Abdominal/Flank/Back Pain, Musculoskeletal Pain (sprains, strains, contusions, fractures, dislocations, subluxations, tendinopathies, arthralgias, back pain)
	Soft Tissue Pain (lacerations, contusions, abscesses)
	Abdominal Migraine Acute/Chronic Neuropathic Pain
	Refractory Migraine Headache
	Vaso-Occlusive Painful Crisis of Sickle Cell Disease
	Opioid-Tolerant Painful Conditions
	Opioid-Induced Hyperalgesic States
	Cancer-Related Pain

(continues)

Opioid Receptor Agonists (Mu-Receptors) (Target Site)	
Medications	**Pain Syndromes**
Morphine **Hydromorphone** **Fentanyl**	Acute Traumatic Musculoskeletal Pain (fractures, dislocations, subluxations)
	Acute Visceral Pain (abdominal pain: biliary colic, pancreatitis, diverticulitis), Renal Colic, Acute Traumatic Pain, Sickle Cell Vaso-Occlusive Painful Crisis, Cancer-Related Pain
TRPV1 Receptor Agonists (Target Site)	
Medications	**Pain Syndromes**
Acetaminophen	Musculoskeletal Pain (sprains, strains, contusions, fractures, dislocations, subluxations, tendinopathies, arthralgias, back pain)
	Soft Tissue Pain (lacerations, contusions, abscesses)
Capsaicin	Musculoskeletal Pain (sprains, strains, contusions)
	Herpetic/Post-Herpetic Neuralgia

(continues)

Volatile Anesthetic (Endogenous Opioid Receptor Agonists) (Target Site)	
Medications	**Pain Syndromes**
Nitrous Oxide	Acute Musculoskeletal Pain (traumatic/non-traumatic): Fractures, Dislocations
	Acute Traumatic/Non-Traumatic Soft Tissue Painful Conditions (lacerations, contusions, abscesses)

ABDOMINAL PAIN (NON-TRAUMATIC)

Inpatient Analgesics (in the ED)	Outpatient Analgesics (discharge)
Non-Opioid	**Non-Opioid**
[1]**IV Ketorolac:** 10–15 mg IVP (analgesic ceiling dose)	[3]**PO Acetaminophen:** 500 mg q8h (max 1500 mg/day based on analgesic ceiling). Best if combined with [5]**Ibuprofen** or [6]**Naproxen**
[2]**IV Lidocaine:** 1.5 mg/kg of 2% (preservative-free lidocaine: cardiac or pre-made bags only) over 15 min (max dose 200 mg)	
[3]**IV Acetaminophen** (APAP): 1 g over 15 min (as adjunct to opioid/non-opioid) if patients are NPO/NPR or contraindications to opioids, NSAIDs, lidocaine, or ketamine	[5]**PO Ibuprofen:** 400 mg q8h × 3 days (max 5 days with 1200 mg/d based on analgesic ceiling)
	[6]**PO Naproxen:** 500 mg q12h × 3 days (max 5 days)
[4]**Ketamine (Subdissociative Dose Ketamine, SDK)**	[7]**PO Diclofenac:** 50 mg q8h × 3 days (max 5 days)
• **IV:** 0.3 mg/kg over 15 min, +/– continuous IV infusion at 0.15–0.2 mg/kg/h	[1]**PO Ketorolac:** 10 mg daily (analgesic ceiling dose; should not be routinely prescribed as ibuprofen and naproxen confer better side effect profile)
• **SQ:** 0.3 mg/kg over 15 min, +/– continuous SQ infusion at 0.15–0.2 mg/kg/h	

(continues)

- **Intranasal (IN):** 0.5–1 mg/kg (weight-based) q5–10 min (consider using highly concentrated solutions:

  Adults: 100 mg/mL

  Peds: 50 mg/mL. No more than 0.3–0.5 mL/per nostril)

Opioid	Opioid
<u>Oral Regimen</u> (for opioid-naïve patients): [8]**Morphine:** Morphine sulfate immediate release (MSIR) 15 mg [9]**Fentanyl:** Transbuccal 100–200 µg dissolvable tablets, repeat at 30–60 min if pain persists [10]**Hydromorphone:** 2 mg <u>Parenteral Regimen</u> (for opioid-naïve patients): [8]**Morphine:** • **IV:** 0.05–0.1 mg/kg (weight-based), titrate q10–20 min • **IV:** 4–6 mg (fixed), titrate q10–20 min • **SQ:** 4–6 mg (fixed), re-administer as needed at q30–40 min	**Oral Opioids** (in order of lesser degree of euphoria): [8]**Morphine Sulfate Immediate Release (MSIR):** 15 mg q6–8h × 2–3 days (opioid-naïve patients) [12]**Hydrocodone/Acetaminophen (Norco):** 5/325 mg: 1–2 tabs q6–8h × 2–3 days [13]**Hydrocodone/Acetaminophen (Vicodin, Lortab, Lorcet):** 5/300 mg: 1–2 tabs q6–8h × 2–3 days [14]**Hydrocodone/Ibuprofen (Vicoprofen):** 5/200 mg: 1–2 tabs q6–8h × 2–3 days [15]**Oxycodone/Acetaminophen (Percocet, Roxicet):** 5/325 mg: 1–2 tabs q4–6h × 2–3 days

(continues)

- **IM:** 4–6 mg (fixed), re-administer as needed at q40–60 min (IM route should be avoided due to pain upon injection, muscle fibrosis, necrosis, increase in dosing requirements)

  Nebulized (via Breath Actuated Nebulizer [BAN]):

  Adults: 10–20 mg (fixed), repeat q15–20 min up to three doses

  Peds: 0.2–0.4 mg/kg (weight-based), repeat q15–20 min up to three doses

- **PCA:**

  Demand dose: 1–2 mg

  Continuous basal infusion: 0.5–2 mg/h

[9]**Fentanyl:**

- **IV:** 0.25–0.5 µg/kg (weight-based), titrate q10 min
- **IV:** 25–50 µg (fixed), titrate q10 min

  Nebulized (via BAN):

[10]**Hydromorphone:** 2 mg q6–8h × 2–3 days (for opioid-naïve patients start with 2 mg dose)

(continues)

Adults: 2–4 µg/kg (weight-based), titrate q20–30 min, up to three doses

Peds: 2–4 µg/kg (weight-based), titrate q20–30 min, up to three doses

- **Intranasal (IN):** 1–2 µg/kg (weight-based), titrate q5–10 min (consider using highly concentrated solutions:

  Adults: 100 µg/mL

  Peds: 50 µg/mL. No more than 0.3–0.5 mL/per nostril)

- **Transmucosal:** 15–20 mcg/kg lollipops

- **PCA:**

  Demand dose: 20–50 µg

  Continuous basal infusion: 0.05–0.1 µg/kg/h

[10]Hydromorphone:

- **IV:** 0.2–0.5 mg initial, titrate q10–15 min

- **SQ:** 0.5–1 mg, titrate q30–40 min

- **IM:** 0.5–1 mg, titrate q30–40 min (IM route should be avoided due to pain, muscle fibrosis, necrosis, increase in dosing requirements)

(continues)

- **PCA:**

   Demand dose: 0.2–0.4 mg

   Continuous basal infusion: 0.1–0.4 mg/h

[11]**Sufentanil:**

- **Intranasal (IN):** 0.5 µg/kg, titration q10 min, up to three doses

---

[1]**KETOROLAC** *(Toradol)*

▶L ☺ ♀B (D in 3rd trimester) ▶+ $$ ■

WARNING – Indicated for short-term (up to 5 days) therapy only. Ketorolac is a potent NSAID and can cause serious GI and renal adverse effects. It may also increase the risk of bleeding by inhibiting platelet function. Contraindicated in patients with active peptic ulcer disease, recent GI bleeding or perforation, a history of peptic ulcer disease or GI bleeding, or advanced renal impairment.

ADULT – Moderately severe, acute pain, single-dose treatment: 30–60 mg IM or 15–30 mg IV. Multiple-dose treatment: 15–30 mg IV/IM q6h. IV/IM doses are not to exceed 60 mg/day for age 65 yo or older, wt < 50 kg, and patients with moderately elevated serum creatinine. Oral continuation therapy: 10 mg PO q4–6h prn, max dose 40 mg/day. Combined duration IV/IM and PO is not to exceed 5 days.

PEDS – Not approved in children.

UNAPPROVED PEDS – Pain: 0.5 mg/kg/dose IM/IV q6h (up to 30 mg q6h or 120 mg/day), give 10 mg PO qGh prn (up to 40 mg/day) for wt > 50 kg.

FORMS – Generic only: Tabs 10 mg.
MOA – Serious: Hypersensitivity, GI bleeding, nephrotoxicity.
Frequent: Nausea, dyspepsia.

[2]LIDOCAINE—LOCAL ANESTHETIC *(Xylocaine)*

▶LK ♀B ▶? $

ADULT – Without epinephrine: Max dose 4.5 mg/kg not to exceed
300 mg. With epinephrine: Max dose 7 mg/kg not to exceed
500 mg. Dose for regional block varies by region.
PEDS – Same as adult.
FORMS – 0.5, 1, 1.5, 2%. With epi: 0.5, 1, 1.5, 2%.
NOTES – Onset within 2 min, duration 30–60 min (longer with
epi). Amide group. Use "cardiac lidocaine" (ie, IV formulation) for Bier blocks at max dose of 3 mg/kg so that neither
epinephrine nor methylparaben is injected IV.
MOA – Amide local anesthetic.
ADVERSE EFFECTS – Serious: Seizures, cardiovascular de-
pression, bradycardia, hypersensitivity, methemoglobinemia.
Frequent: None.

[3]ACETAMINOPHEN *(Tylenol, Panadol, Tempra, Ofirmev, Paracetamol, Abenol, Atasol, Pediatrix)*

▶LK ♀B ▶+ $

ADULT – Analgesic/antipyretic: 325–1000 mg PO q4–6h prn.
650 mg PR q4–6h prn. Max dose 4 g/day. OA: Extended-release:
2 caps PO q8h around the clock. Max dose 6 caps/day.
PEDS – Analgesic/antipyretic: 10–15 mg/kg q4–6h PO/PR
prn. Max 5 doses/day.
UNAPPROVED ADULT – OA: 1000 mg PO four times per day.

FORMS – OTC: Tabs 325, 500, 650 mg. Chewable tabs 80 mg. Orally disintegrating tabs 80, 160 mg. Caps/gelcaps 500 mg. Extended-release caplets 650 mg. Liquid 160 mg/5 mL, 500 mg/15 mL. Supps 80, 120, 325, 650 mg.

NOTES – Risk of hepatotoxicity with chronic use, especially in alcoholics. Caution in those who drink three or more drinks/day. Rectal administration may produce lower/less reliable plasma levels.

MOA – Analgesic/antipyretic.

ADVERSE EFFECTS – Serious: Hepatotoxicity. Frequent: None.

[4]KETAMINE *(Ketalar)*

▶L ♀C ▶? ©III $ ■

WARNING – Post-anesthetic emergence reactions up to 24 h later manifested as dreamlike state, vivid imagery, hallucinations, and delirium reported in about 12% of cases. Incidence reduced when (1) age less than 15 yo or greater than 65 yo, (2) concomitant use of benzodiazepines, lower dose, or used as induction agent only (because of use of post-intubation sedation).

ADULT – Induction of anesthesia: Adult: 1–2 mg/kg IV over 1–2 min (produces 5–10 min dissociative state) or 6.5–13 mg/kg IM (produces 10–20 min dissociative state).

PEDS – Age over 16 yo: same as adult.

UNAPPROVED ADULT – Dissociative sedation: 1–2 mg/kg IV over 1–2 mm (sedation lasting 10–20 min) repeat 0.5 mg/kg doses every 5–15 min may be given; 4–5 mg/kg IM (sedation lasting 15–30 min) repeat 2–4 mg/kg IM can be given if needed after 10–15 min. Analgesia adjunct subdissociative dose: 0.01–0.5 mg/kg in conjunction with opioid analgesia.

UNAPPROVED PEDS — Dissociative sedation: Age older than 3 mo: 1–2 mg/kg IV (produces 5–10 min dissociative state) over 1–2 min or 4–5 mg/kg IM (produces 10–20 min dissociative state). Not approved for age younger than 3 mo.

FORMS — Generic/Trade: 10, 50, 100 mg/mL.

NOTES — Recent evidence suggests ketamine is not contraindicated in patients with head injuries. However, avoid if CAD or severe HTN. Concurrent administration of atropine no longer recommended. Consider prophylactic ondansetron to reduce vomiting and prophylactic midazolam (0.3 mg/kg) to reduce recovery reactions.

MOA — NMDA receptor antagonist which produces dissociative state.

ADVERSE EFFECTS — Serious: Laryngospasm, hallucinatory emergence reactions, hypersalivation. Frequent: Nystagmus, hypertension, tachycardia, N/V, muscular hypertonicity, myoclonus.

[5]IBUPROFEN *(Motrin, Advil, Nuprin, Rufen, NeoProfen, Caldolor)*

▶L ⊗ ♀B (D in 3rd trimester) ▶+ ■

ADULT — RA/OA, gout: 200–800 mg PO three to four times per day. Mild to moderate pain: 400 mg PO q4–6h. 400–800 mg IV (Caldolor) q6h prn. 400 mg IV (Caldolor) q4–6h or 100–200 mg q4h prn. Primary dysmenorrhea: 400 mg PO q4h prn. Fever: 200 mg PO q4–6h prn. Migraine pain: 200–400 mg PO not to exceed 400 mg in 24 h unless directed by a physician (OTC dosing). Max dose 3.2 g/day.

PEDS — JRA: 30–50 mg/kg/day PO divided q6h. Max dose 2400 mg/24 h. 20 mg/kg/day may be adequate for milder disease. Analgesic/antipyretic, age older than 6 mo: 5–10 mg/kg

PO q6–8h, prn. Max dose 40 mg/kg/day. Patent ductus arteriosus in neonates 32 weeks' gestational age or younger weighing 500–1500 g (NeoProfen): Specialized dosing.

FORMS – OTC: Caps/Liqui-Gel caps 200 mg. Tabs 100, 200 mg. Chewable tabs 100 mg. Susp (infant gtts) 50 mg/1.25 mL (with calibrated dropper), 100 mg/5 mL. Rx Generic/Trade: Tabs 400, 600, 800 mg.

NOTES – May antagonize antiplatelet effects of aspirin if given simultaneously. Take aspirin 2 h prior to ibuprofen. Administer IV (Caldolor) over at least 30 min; hydration important.

MOA – Anti-inflammatory/antipyretic, analgesic.

ADVERSE EFFECTS – Serious: Hypersensitivity, GI bleeding, nephrotoxicity. Frequent: Nausea, dyspepsia.

[6]NAPROXEN (Naprosyn, Aleve, Anaprox, EC-Naprosyn, Naprelan, Prevacid, NapraPAC)

▶L ☒ ♀B (D in 3rd trimester) ▶+ $ ■

WARNING – Multiple strengths; see FORMS and write specific product on Rx.

ADULT – RA/OA, ankylosing spondylitis, pain, dysmenorrhea, acute tendinitis and bursitis, fever: 250–500 mg PO two times per day. Delayed-release: 375–500 mg PO two times per day (do not crush or chew). Controlled-release: 750–1000 mg PO daily. Acute gout: 750 mg PO once, then 250 mg PO q8h until the attack subsides. Controlled-release: 1000–1500 mg PO once, then 1000 mg PO daily until the attack subsides.

PEDS – JRA: 10–20 mg/kg/day PO divided two times per day (up to 1250 mg/24 h). Pain for age older than 2 yo: 5–7 mg/kg/dose PO q8–12 h.

UNAPPROVED ADULT — Acute migraine: 750 mg PO once, then 250–500 mg PO prn. Migraine prophylaxis, menstrual migraine: 500 mg PO two times per day beginning 1 day prior to onset of menses and ending on last day of period.

FORMS — OTC Generic/Trade (Aleve): Tabs, immediate-release 200 mg. OTC Trade only (Aleve): Caps, Gelcaps, immediate-release 200 mg. Rx Generic/Trade: Tabs, immediate-release (Naprosyn) 250, 375, 500 mg. (Anaprox) 275, 550 mg. Tabs, delayed-release enteric-coated (EC-Naprosyn) 375, 500 mg. Tabs, controlled-release (Naprelan) 375, 500, 750 mg. Susp (Naprosyn) 125 mg/5 mL. Prevacid NapraPAC: 7 lansoprazole 15-mg caps packaged with 14 naproxen tabs 375 mg or 500 mg.

NOTES — All dosing is based on naproxen content: 500 mg naproxen is equivalent to 550 mg naproxen sodium.

MOA — Anti-inflammatory, analgesic.

ADVERSE EFFECTS — Serious: Hypersensitivity, GI bleeding, nephrotoxicity. Frequent: Nausea, dyspepsia.

---

[7]**DICLOFENAC (Voltaren, Voltaren XR, Flector, Zipsor, Cambia, Zorvolex, Voltaren Rapide)**

▶L ⊗ ♀B (D in 3rd trimester) ▶– $$$

WARNING — Multiple strengths; see FORMS and write specific product on Rx.

ADULT — OA: Immediate- or delayed-release: 50 mg PO two to three times per day or 75 mg two times per day. Extended-release 100 mg PO daily. Gel: Apply 4 g to knees or 2 g to hands four times per day using enclosed dosing card. RA: Immediate- or delayed-release 50 mg PO three to four times per day or 75 mg two times per day. Extended-release 100 mg PO one to two times per day. Ankylosing spondylitis: Immediate- or delayed-release 25 mg PO four times per day and at bedtime. Analgesia and primary dysmenorrhea: Immediate- or delayed-release 50 mg PO three times per day. Acute pain in strains, sprains, or contusions: Apply 1 patch to painful area two times per day. Acute migraine with or without aura: 50 mg single dose (Cambia), mix packet with 30–60 mL water.

PEDS – Not approved in children.

UNAPPROVED PEDS – JRA: 2–3 mg/kg/day PO.

FORMS – Generic/Trade: Tabs, extended-release (Voltaren XR) 100 mg. Topical gel (Voltaren) 1% 100 g tube. Generic only: Tabs, immediate-release: 25, 50 mg. Generic only: Tabs, delayed-release: 25, 50, 75 mg. Trade only: Patch (Flector) 1.3% diclofenac epolamine. Trade only: Caps, liquid-filled (Zipsor) 25 mg. Caps (Zorvolex) 18, 35 mg. Trade only: Powder for oral soln (Cambia) 50 mg.

NOTES – Check LFTs at baseline, within 4–8 weeks of initiation, then periodically. Do not apply patch to damaged or nonintact skin. Wash hands, and avoid eye contact when handling the patch. Do not wear patch while bathing or showering.

MOA – Anti-inflammatory, analgesic.

ADVERSE EFFECTS – Serious: Hypersensitivity, GI bleeding, hepato/nephrotoxicity. Frequent: Nausea, dyspepsia, pruritus, and dermatitis with patch and gel.

[8]**MORPHINE** *(MS Contin, Kadian, Avinza, Roxanol, Oramorph SR, MSIR, DepoDur, Statex, M.O.S. Doloral, M-Eslon)*

▶LK ⊗ ♀C ▶+ ©II Varies by therapy ■

WARNING – Multiple strengths; see FORMS and write specific product on Rx. Drinking alcohol while taking

Avinza may result in a rapid release of a potentially fatal dose of morphine.

ADULT – Moderate to severe pain: 10–30 mg PO q4h (immediate-release tabs, or oral soln). Controlled-release (MS Contin, Oramorph SR): 30 mg PO q8–12h. (Kadian): 20 mg PO q12–24h. Extended-release caps (Avinza): 30 mg PO daily. 10 mg q4h IM/SC. 2.5–15 mg/70 kg IV over 4–5 min. 10–20 mg PR q4h. Pain with major surgery (DepoDur): 10–15 mg once epidurally at the lumbar level prior to surgery (max dose 20 mg), or 10 mg epidurally after clamping of the umbilical cord with cesarean section.

PEDS – Moderate to severe pain: 0.1–0.2 mg/kg up to 15 mg IM/SC/IV q2–4h.

UNAPPROVED PEDS – Moderate to severe pain: 0.2–0.5 mg/kg/dose PO (immediate-release) q4–6h. 0.3–0.6 mg/kg/dose PO (controlled-release) q12h.

FORMS – Generic only: Tabs, immediate-release 15, 30 mg ($). Oral soln 10 mg/5 mL, 20 mg/5 mL, 20 mg/mL (concentrate). Rectal supps 5, 10, 20, 30 mg. Generic/Trade: Controlled-release tabs (MS Contin) 15, 30, 60, 100, 200 mg ($$$$). Controlled-release caps (Kadian) 10, 20, 30, 50, 60, 80, 100 mg ($$$$$). Extended-release caps (Avinza) 30, 45, 60, 75, 90, 120 mg. Trade only: Controlled-release caps (Kadian) 40, 200 mg.

NOTES – Titrate dose as high as necessary to relieve cancer or nonmalignant pain where chronic opioids are necessary. The active metabolites may accumulate in hepatic/renal insufficiency and the elderly leading to increased analgesic and sedative effects. Do not break, chew, or crush MS Contin or Oramorph SR. Kadian and Avinza caps may be opened and sprinkled in applesauce for easier administration; however, the pellets should not be crushed or chewed. Doses more than 1600 mg/day of Avinza contain a potentially nephrotoxic quantity of fumaric acid. Do not mix DepoDur with other medications; do not administer any other medications into epidural space for at least 48 h. Severe opiate overdose with respiratory depression has occurred with intrathecal leakage of DepoDur.

MOA — Opioid agonist analgesic.

ADVERSE EFFECTS — Serious: Respiratory depression/arrest. Frequent: N/V, constipation, sedation, hypotension.

[9]FENTANYL *(IONSYS, Duragesic, Actiq, Fentora, Sublimaze, Abstral, Subsys, Lazanda, Onsolis)*

▶L ⊗ ♀C ▶+ ©II Varies by therapy ■

WARNING — Duragesic patches, Actiq, Fentora, Abstral, Subsys, and Lazanda are contraindicated in the management of acute or postop pain due to potentially life-threatening respiratory depression in opioid nontolerant patients. Instruct patients and their caregivers that even used patches/lozenges on a stick can be fatal to a child or pet. Dispose via toilet. Actiq and Fentora are not interchangeable. IONSYS: For hospital use only; remove prior to discharge. Can cause life-threatening respiratory depression.

ADULT — Duragesic patches: Chronic pain: 12–100 mcg/h patch q72h. Titrate dose to the needs of the patient. Some patients require q48h dosing. May wear more than 1 patch to achieve the correct analgesic effect. Actiq: Breakthrough cancer pain: 200–1600 mcg sucked over 15 min; if 200 mcg ineffective for 6 units use higher strength. Goal is 4 lozenges on a stick/day in conjunction with long-acting opioid. Buccal tab (Fentora) for breakthrough cancer pain: 100–800 mcg, titrated to pain relief; may repeat once after 30 min during single episode of breakthrough pain. See prescribing information for dose conversion from transmucosal lozenges. Buccal soluble film (Onsolis) for breakthrough cancer pain: 200–1200 mcg titrated to pain relief; no more than 4 doses/day separated by at least 2 h. Postop analgesia: 50–100 mcg IM; repeat in 1–2 h prn. SL tab (Abstral) for breakthrough cancer pain: 100 mcg, may repeat once after 30 min. Specialized titration. SL spray (Subsys) for breakthrough cancer pain 100 mcg, may repeat once after 30 min. Specialized titration. Nasal spray (Lazanda) for breakthrough cancer pain: 100 mcg. Specialized titration. IONSYS: Acute postop pain: Specialized dosing.

PEDS — Transdermal (Duragesic): Not approved in children younger than 2 yo or in opioid-naïve. Use adult dosing for age older than 2 yo. Children converting to a 25-mcg patch should be receiving 45 mg or more oral morphine equivalents/day. Actiq: Not approved for age younger than 16 yo. IONSYS not approved in children. Abstral, Subsys, and Lazanda: Not approved for age younger than 18 yo.

UNAPPROVED ADULT — Analgesia/procedural sedation/labor analgesia: 50–100 mcg IV or IM q1–2h prn.

UNAPPROVED PEDS — Analgesia: 1–2 mcg/kg/dose IV/IM q30–60 min prn or continuous IV infusion 1–3 mcg/kg/h (not to exceed adult dosing). Procedural sedation: 2–3 mcg/kg/dose for age 1–3 yo; 1–2 mcg/kg/dose for age 3–12 yo, 0.5–1 mcg/kg/dose (not to exceed adult dosing) for age older than 12 yo, procedural sedation doses may be repeated q30–60 min prn.

FORMS — Generic/Trade: Transdermal patches 12, 25, 50, 75, 100 mcg/h. Actiq lozenges on a stick, berry-flavored 200, 400, 600, 800, 1200, 1600 mcg. Trade only: (Fentora) buccal tab

100, 200, 400, 600, 800 mcg, packs of 4 or 28 tabs. Trade only: (Onsolis) buccal soluble film 200, 400, 600, 800, 1200 mcg in child-resistant, protective foil, packs of 30 films. Trade only: (Abstral) SL tabs 100, 200, 300, 400, 600, 800 mcg, packs of 4 or 32 tabs. Trade only: (Subsys) SL spray 100, 200, 400, 600, 800, 1200, 1600 mcg blister packs in cartons of 10 and 30 (30 only for 1200 and 1600 mcg). Trade only: (Lazanda) nasal spray 100, 400 mcg/spray, 8 sprays/bottle.

NOTES — Do not use patches for acute pain or in opioid-naïve patients. Oral transmucosal fentanyl doses of 5 mcg/kg provide effects similar to 0.75–1.25 mcg/kg of fentanyl IM. Lozenges on a stick should be sucked, not chewed. Flush lozenge remnants (without stick) down the toilet. For transdermal systems: Apply patch to non-hairy skin. Clip (do not shave) hair if you have to apply to hairy area. Fever or external heat sources may increase fentanyl released from patch. Patch should be removed prior to MRI and reapplied after the test. Dispose of a used patch by folding with the adhesive side of the patch adhering to itself then flush it down the toilet immediately. Do not cut the patch in half. For Duragesic patches and Actiq lozenges on a stick: Titrate dose as high as necessary to relieve cancer or nonmalignant pain where chronic opioids are necessary. Do not suck, chew, or swallow buccal tab. IONSYS: Apply to intact skin on the chest or upper arm. Each dose activated by the patient is delivered over a 10-min period. Remove prior to hospital discharge. Do not allow gel to touch mucous membranes. Dispose using gloves. Keep all forms of fentanyl out of the reach of children or pets. Concomitant use with potent CYP3A4 inhibitors such as ritonavir, ketoconazole, itraconazole, clarithromycin, nelfinavir, and nefazodone may result in an increase in fentanyl plasma concentrations, which could increase or prolong adverse drug effects and may cause potentially fatal respiratory depression. Onsolis is available only through the FOCUS Program and requires prescriber, pharmacy, and patient enrollment. Used films should be discarded into toilet. Abstral, Subsys, and Lazanda: Outpatients, prescribers, pharmacies, and distributors must be enrolled in TIRF REMS Access program before patient may receive medication.

MOA – Opioid agonist analgesic.

ADVERSE EFFECTS – Serious: Respiratory depression/arrest, chest wall rigidity. Frequent: N/V, constipation, sedation, skin irritation, dental decay with Actiq.

[10]HYDROMORPHONE *(Dilaudid, Exalgo, Hydromorph Contin)*

▶L ⊗ ♀C ▷? ©‖ $$ ■

ADULT – Moderate to severe pain: 2–4 mg PO q4–6h. Initial dose (opioid-naïve): 0.5–2 mg SC/IM or slow IV q4–6h prn. 3 mg PR q6–8h. Controlled-release tabs: 8–64 mg daily.

PEDS – Not approved in children.

UNAPPROVED PEDS – Pain age 12 yo or younger: 0.03–0.08 mg/kg PO q4–6h prn. 0.015 mg/kg/dose IV q4–6h prn, use adult dose for older than 12 yo.

FORMS – Generic/Trade: Tabs 2, 4, 8 mg (8 mg trade scored). Oral soln 5 mg/5 mL. Controlled-release tabs (Exalgo): 8, 12, 16, 32 mg.

NOTES – In opioid-naïve patients, consider an initial dose of 0.5 mg or less IM/SC/IV/. SC/IM/IV doses after initial dose should be individualized. May be given by slow IV injection over

2–5 min. Titrate dose as high as necessary to relieve cancer or nonmalignant pain where chronic opioids are necessary. 1.5 mg IV = 7.5 mg PO. Exalgo intended for opioid-tolerant patients only.

MOA – Opioid agonist analgesic.

ADVERSE EFFECTS – Serious: Respiratory depression/arrest. Frequent: N/V, constipation, sedation.

[11]SUFENTANIL (Sufenta)

▶L ♀C ▶? ©II $$

ADULT – General anesthesia: Induction: 8–30 mcg/kg IV; maintenance 0.5–10 mcg/kg IV. Conscious sedation: Loading dose: 0.1–0.5 mcg/kg; maintenance infusion 0.005–0.01 mcg/kg/min.

PEDS – General anesthesia: Induction: 8–30 mcg/kg IV; maintenance 0.5–10 mcg/kg IV. Conscious sedation: Loading dose: 0.1–0.5 mcg/kg; maintenance infusion 0.005–0.01 mcg/kg/min.

MOA – Serious: Respiratory depression, hypotension, bradycardia, chest wall rigidity, opiate dependence, hypersensitivity. Frequent: Sedation, N/V.

[12]NORCO (hydrocodone + acetaminophen)

▶L ⊗ ♀C ▶? ©II $$

WARNING – Multiple strengths; see FORMS and write specific product on Rx.

ADULT – Moderate to severe pain: 1–2 tabs PO q4–6h prn (5/325), max dose 12 tabs/day. 1 tab (7.5/325 and 10/325) PO q4–6h prn, max dose 8 and 6 tabs/day, respectively.

PEDS – Not approved in children.

FORMS – Generic/Trade: Tabs 5/325, 7.5/325, 10/325 mg hydrocodone/acetaminophen, scored. Generic only: Soln 7.5/325 mg per 15 mL.

[13]VICODIN *(hydrocodone + acetaminophen)*

▶LK ✪ ♀C ▶? ⊚II $$$

WARNING – Multiple strengths; see FORMS and write specific product on Rx.

ADULT – Moderate pain: 5/300 mg (max dose 8 tabs/day) and 7.5/300 mg (max dose of 6 tabs/day): 1–2 tabs PO q4–6h prn. 10/300 mg: 1 tab PO q4–6h prn (max of 6 tabs/day).

PEDS – Not approved in children.

FORMS – Generic/Trade: Tabs Vicodin (5/300), Vicodin ES (7.5/300), Vicodin HP (10/300) mg hydrocodone/mg acetaminophen, scored.

[13]LORTAB *(hydrocodone + acetaminophen)*

▶LK ✪ ♀C ▶– ⊚II $$

WARNING – Multiple strengths; see FORMS and write specific product on Rx.

ADULT – Moderate pain: 1–2 tabs 2.5/325 and 5/325 PO q4–6h prn, max dose 8 tabs/day. 1 tab 7.5/325 and 10/325 PO q4–6h prn, max dose 5 tabs/day.

PEDS – Not approved in children.

FORMS – Generic/Trade: Lortab 5/325 (scored), Lortab 7.5/325 (trade scored), Lortab 10/325 mg hydrocodone/mg acetaminophen. Generic only: Tabs 2.5/325 mg.

MOA – Serious: Respiratory depression/arrest, hepatotoxicity. Frequent: N/V, constipation, sedation.

[13]LORCET *(hydrocodone + acetaminophen)*

▶LK ⊗ ♀C ▶– ⊚II $$

WARNING – Multiple strengths; see FORMS and write specific product on Rx.

ADULT – Moderate pain: 1–2 caps (5/325) PO q4–6h prn, max dose 8 caps/day. 1 tab PO q4–6h prn (7.5/325 and 10/325), max dose 6 tabs/day.

PEDS – Not approved in children.

FORMS – Generic/Trade: Tabs, 5/325, 7.5/325, 10/325 mg.

[14]VICOPROFEN *(hydrocodone + ibuprofen)*

▶LK ⊗ ♀– ▶? ⊚II $$

ADULT – Moderate pain: 1 tab PO q4–6h prn, max dose 5 tabs/day.

PEDS – Not approved in children.

FORMS – Generic only: Tabs 2.5/200, 5/200, 10/200 mg hydrocodone/ibuprofen.

NOTES – See NSAIDs—Other subclass warning.

MOA – Combination analgesic.

ADVERSE EFFECTS – Serious: Respiratory depression/arrest, hypersensitivity, GI bleeding, nephrotoxicity. Frequent: N/V, constipation, dyspepsia, sedation.

[15]PERCOCET *(oxycodone + acetaminophen, Percocet-Demi, Oxycocet, Endocet)*

▶L ⊗ ♀C ▶– ⊚II $

WARNING – Multiple strengths; see FORMS and write specific product on Rx.

ADULT – Moderate to severe pain: 1–2 tabs PO q4–6h prn (2.5/325 and 5/325 mg). 1 tab PO q4–6h prn (7.5/325 and 10/325 mg).

PEDS – Not approved in children.

FORMS – Generic/Trade: Oxycodone/acetaminophen tabs 2.5/325, 5/325, 7.5/325, 10/325 mg. Trade only: (Primlev) tabs 2.5/300, 5/300, 7.5/300, 10/300 mg. Generic only: 10/325 mg.

[15]ROXICET *(oxycodone + acetaminophen)*

▶L ⊗ ♀C ▶– ©II $

WARNING – Multiple strengths; see FORMS and write specific product on Rx.

ADULT – Moderate to severe pain: 1 tab PO q6h prn. Oral soln: 5 mL PO q6h prn.

PEDS – Not approved in children.

FORMS – Generic/Trade: Tabs 5/325 mg. Caps/caplets 5/325 mg. Soln 5/325 per 5 mL mg oxycodone/acetaminophen.

ABDOMINAL PAIN (TRAUMATIC)

Inpatient Analgesics (in the ED)	Outpatient Analgesics (discharge)
Non-Opioid	**Non-Opioid**
[1]**IV Lidocaine:** 1.5 mg/kg of 2% (preservative-free lidocaine-cardiac or pre-made bags only) over 15 min (max dose 200 mg)	[2]**PO Acetaminophen:** 500 mg q8h (max 1500 mg/day based on analgesic ceiling). Best if combined with [6]**Ibuprofen** or naproxen
[2]**IV Acetaminophen (APAP):** 1 g over 15 min (as adjunct to opioid/non-opioid) if patients are NPO/NPR or contraindications to opioids, NSAIDs, lidocaine, or ketamine	[6]**PO Ibuprofen:** 400 mg q8h × 3 days (max 5 days with 1200 mg/d based on analgesic ceiling)
[3]**Ketamine (Subdissociative Dose Ketamine, SDK)**	[7]**PO Naproxen:** 500 mg q12h × 3 days (max 5 days)
• **IV:** 0.3 mg/kg over 15 min, +/− continuous IV infusion at 0.15–0.2 mg/kg/h	[8]**PO Diclofenac:** 50 mg q8h × 3 days (max 5 days)
• **SQ:** 0.3 mg/kg over 15 min, +/− continuous SQ infusion at 0.15–0.2 mg/kg/h	[9]**PO Ketorolac:** 10 mg daily (analgesic ceiling dose, should not be routinely prescribed as ibuprofen and naproxen confer better side effect profile)
• **Intranasal (IN):** 0.5–1 mg/kg (weight-based) q5–10 min (consider using highly concentrated solutions: Adults: 100 mg/mL Peds: 50 mg/mL. No more than 0.3–0.5 mL/per nostril)	[10]**Topical NSAIDs** (Diclofenac Cream, Patch) for abdominal wall trauma
	[11]**Topical Lidocaine** 4–5% patch, 2% cream) for abdominal wall trauma

(continues)

IV Ketorolac: 10–15 mg IVP (analgesic ceiling dose) (abdominal wall contusions, superficial penetrating trauma, blunt trauma)

Regional Block (UGRA) for abdominal wall injuries: Transversus Abdominis Plane (TAP) Block

[4]**Bupivacaine w/o Epinephrine:** 0.25–0.5%, max 2.5 mg/kg

[4]**Bupivacaine w/ Epinephrine:** 0.25–0.5%, max 3.0 mg/kg

[1]**Lidocaine w/o Epinephrine:** 0.5–2%, 4.5 mg/kg, max 300 mg

[1]**Lidocaine w/ Epinephrine:** 0.5–2%, 7 mg/kg, max 500 mg

[5]**Chloroprocaine:** 2–3%, max 11 mg/kg

[12]**Topical Capsaicin (0.025–0.15% cream)** for abdominal wall trauma

Opioid	Opioid
<u>Oral Regimen</u> (for opioid-naïve patients): [13]**Morphine:** Morphine Sulfate Immediate Release (MSIR): 15 mg [14]**Fentanyl:** Transbuccal 100–200 µg dissolvable tablets, repeat at 30–60 min if pain persists [15]**Hydromorphone:** 2 mg	**Oral Opioids** (in order of lesser degree of euphoria): [12]**Morphine Sulfate Immediate Release (MSIR):** 15 mg q6–8h × 2–3 days (opioid-naïve patients) [17]**Hydrocodone/Acetaminophen (Norco):** 5/325 mg: 1–2 tabs q6–8h × 2–3 days

(*continues*)

<u>**Parenteral Regimen (for opioid-naïve patients):**</u>

[13]Morphine:

- **IV:** 0.05–0.1 mg/kg (weight-based), titrate q10–20 min
- **IV:** 4–6 mg (fixed), titrate q10–20 min
- **SQ:** 4–6 mg (fixed), re-administer as needed at q30–40 min
- **IM:** 4–6 mg (fixed), re-administer as needed at q30–40 min (IM route should be avoided due to pain upon injection, muscle fibrosis, necrosis, increase in dosing requirements)

  Nebulized (via Breath Actuated Nebulizer [BAN]):

  Adults: 10–20 mg (fixed), repeat q15–20 min up to three doses

  Peds: 0.2–0.4 mg/kg (weight-based), repeat q15–20 min up to three doses

- **PCA:**

  Demand dose: 1–2 mg

  Continuous basal infusion: 0.5–2 mg/h

[18]Hydrocodone/ Acetaminophen (Vicodin, Lortab, Lorcet) 5/300 mg: 1–2 tabs q6–8h × 2–3 days

[19]Hydrocodone/Ibuprofen (Vicoprofen) 5/200 mg: 1–2 tabs q6–8h × 2–3 days

[20]Oxycodone/Acetaminophen (Percocet, Roxicet) 5/325 mg: 1–2 tabs q6–8h × 2–3 days

[15]Hydromorphone: 2–4 mg q6–8h × 2–3 days (for opioid-naïve patients start with 2 mg dose)

(*continues*)

[14]**Fentanyl:**

- **IV:** 0.25–0.5 µg/kg (weight-based), titrate q10 min
- **IV:** 25–50 µg (fixed), titrate q10 min

  Nebulized (via BAN):

  Adults: 2–4 µg/kg (weight-based), titrate q20–30 min, up to three doses

  Peds: 2–4 µg/kg (weight-based), titrate q20–30 min, up to three doses

- **Intranasal (IN):** 1–2 µg/kg (weight-based), titrate q5–10 min (consider using highly concentrated solutions:

  Adults: 100 µg/mL

  Peds: 50 µg/mL. No more than 0.3–0.5 mL/per nostril)

- **Transmucosal:** 15–20 mcg/kg lollipops
- **PCA:**

  Demand dose: 20–50 µg

  Continuous basal infusion: 0.05-0.1 µg/kg/h

(*continues*)

[15]**Hydromorphone:**
- **IV:** 0.2–0.5 mg initial, titrate q10–15 min
- **SQ:** 0.5–1 mg, titrate q30–40 min
- **IM:** 0.5–1 mg, titrate q30–40 min (IM route should be avoided due to pain, muscle fibrosis, necrosis, increase in dosing requirements)
- **PCA:**

  Demand dose: 0.2–0.4 mg

  Continuous basal infusion: 0.1–0.4 mg/h

[16]**Sufentanil:**
- **Intranasal (IN):** 0.5 µg/kg, titration q10 min up to three doses

KETOROLAC (Toradol)

▶L ⊗ ♀C (D in 3rd trimester) ▶+ $$ ■

WARNING – Indicated for short-term (up to 5 days) therapy only. Ketorolac is a potent NSAID and can cause serious GI and renal adverse effects. It may also increase the risk of bleeding by inhibiting platelet function. Contraindicated in patients with active peptic ulcer disease, recent GI bleeding or perforation, a history of peptic ulcer disease or GI bleeding, or advanced renal impairment.

ADULT – Moderately severe, acute pain, single-dose treatment: 30–60 mg IM or 15–30 mg IV. Multiple-dose treatment: 15–30 mg IV/IM q6 h. IV/IM doses are not to exceed 60 mg/day for age 65 yo or older, wt, 50 kg, and patients with moderately elevated serum creatinine. Oral continuation therapy: 10 mg PO q4–6h prn, max dose 40 mg/day. Combined duration IV/IM and PO is not to exceed 5 days.

PEDS – Not approved in children.

UNAPPROVED PEDS – Pain: 0.5 mg/kg/dose IM/IV q6h (up to 30 mg q6h or 120 mg/day), give 10 mg PO qGh pm (up to 40 mg/day) for wt .50 kg.

[1]LIDOCAINE—LOCAL ANESTHETIC *(Xylocaine)*

▶LK ♀B ▶? $

ADULT – Without epinephrine: Max dose 4.5 mg/kg not to exceed 300 mg. With epinephrine: Max dose 7 mg/kg not to exceed 500 mg. Dose for regional block varies by region.

PEDS – Same as adult.

FORMS – 0.5, 1, 1.5, 2%. With epi: 0.5, 1, 1.5, 2%.

NOTES – Onset within 2 min, duration 30–60 min (longer with epi). Amide group. Use "cardiac lidocaine" (ie, IV formulation) for Bier blocks at max dose of 3 mg/kg so that neither epinephrine nor methylparaben is injected IV.

MOA – Amide local anesthetic.

ADVERSE EFFECTS – Serious: Seizures, cardiovascular depression, bradycardia, hypersensitivity, methemoglobinemia. Frequent: None.

[2]ACETAMINOPHEN *(Tylenol, Panadol, Tempra, Ofirmev, Paracetamol, Abenol, Atasol, Pediatrix)*

▶LK ♀B ▶+ $

ADULT – Analgesic/antipyretic: 325–1000 mg PO q4–6h pm. 650 mg PR q4–6h pm. Max dose 4 g/day. OA: Extended-release: 2 caps PO q8h around the clock. Max dose 6 caps/day.

PEDS – Analgesic/antipyretic: 10–15 mg/kg q4–6h PO/PR pm. Max 5 doses/day.

UNAPPROVED ADULT – OA: 1000 mg PO four times per day.

FORMS – OTC: Tabs 325, 500, 650 mg. Chewable tabs 80 mg. Orally disintegrating tabs 80, 160 mg. Caps/gelcaps 500 mg. Extended-release caplets 650 mg. Liquid 160 mg/5 mL, 500 mg/15 mL. Supps 80, 120, 325, 650 mg.

NOTES – Risk of hepatotoxicity with chronic use, especially in alcoholics. Caution in those who drink three or more drinks/day. Rectal administration may produce lower/less reliable plasma levels.

MOA – Analgesic/antipyretic.

ADVERSE EFFECTS – Serious: Hepatotoxicity. Frequent: None.

[3]KETAMINE *(Ketalar)*

▶L ♀C ▶? ©III $ ■

WARNING – Post-anesthetic emergence reactions up to 24 h later manifested as dreamlike state, vivid imagery, hallucinations, and delirium reported in about 12% of cases. Incidence reduced when (1) age less than 15 yo or greater than 65 yo, (2) concomitant use of benzodiazepines, lower dose, or used as induction agent only (because of use of post-intubation sedation).

ADULT — Induction of anesthesia: Adult: 1–2 mg/kg IV over 1–2 min (produces 5–10 min dissociative state) or 6.5–13 mg/kg IM (produces 10–20 min dissociative state).

PEDS — Age over 16 yo: same as adult.

UNAPPROVED ADULT — Dissociative sedation: 1–2 mg/kg IV over 1–2 mm (sedation lasting 10–20 min) repeat 0.5 mg/kg doses every 5–15 min may be given; 4–5 mg/kg IM (sedation lasting 15–30 min) repeat 2–4 mg/kg IM can be given if needed after 10–15 min. Analgesia adjunct subdissociative dose: 0.01–0.5 mg/kg in conjunction with opioid analgesia.

UNAPPROVED PEDS — Dissociative sedation: Age older than 3 mo: 1–2 mg/kg IV (produces 5–10 min dissociative state) over 1–2 min or 4–5 mg/kg IM (produces 10–20 min dissociative state). Not approved for age younger than 3 mo.

FORMS — Generic/Trade: 10, 50, 100 mg/mL.

NOTES — Recent evidence suggests ketamine is not contraindicated in patients with head injuries. However, avoid if CAD or severe HTN. Concurrent administration of atropine no longer recommended. Consider prophylactic ondansetron to reduce vomiting and prophylactic midazolam (0.3 mg/kg) to reduce recovery reactions.

MOA — NMDA receptor antagonist that produces a dissociative state.

ADVERSE EFFECTS — Serious: Laryngospasm, hallucinatory emergence reactions, hypersalivation. Frequent: Nystagmus, hypertension, tachycardia, N/V, muscular hypertonicity, myoclonus.

[4]BUPIVACAINE *(Marcaine, Sensorcaine)*

▶LK ♀C ▶? $ ■

ADULT – Local anesthesia, nerve block: 0.25% injection. Up to 2.5 mg/kg without epinephrine and up 3.0 mg/kg with epinephrine.

PEDS – Not recommended in children younger than 12 yo.

FORMS – 0.25%, 0.5%, 0.75%, all with or without epinephrine.

NOTES – Onset 5 min, duration 2–4 h (longer with epi). Amide group.

MOA – Amide local anesthetic.

ADVERSE EFFECTS – Serious: Seizures, cardiovascular depression, bradycardia, hypersensitivity, methemoglobinemia. Frequent: None.

[5]CHLOROPROCAINE *(Nesacaine)*

▶LK ♀C ▶? $

ADULT – Epidural anesthesia: 18–24 mL of 2.0–3.0% chloroprocaine will provide 30–60 min of surgical anesthesia. Infiltration and peripheral nerve block: 0.5–40 mL of 1–3% chloroprocaine.

PEDS – Same as adult, age 3 yo or older.

FORMS – 1, 2, 3%.

NOTES – Max local dose: 11 mg/kg.

MOA – Ester local anesthetic.

ADVERSE EFFECTS – Serious: Seizures, cardiovascular depression, bradycardia, hypersensitivity, methemoglobinemia. Frequent: None.

[6]IBUPROFEN *(Motrin, Advil, Nuprin, Rufen, NeoProfen, Caldolor)*

▶L ⊘ ♀B (D in 3rd trimester) ▶+ ■

ADULT — RA/OA, gout: 200–800 mg PO three to four times per day. Mild to moderate pain: 400 mg PO q4–6h. 400–800 mg IV (Caldolor) q6h prn. 400 mg IV (Caldolor) q4–6h or 100–200 mg q4h prn. Primary dysmenorrhea: 400 mg PO q4h prn. Fever: 200 mg PO q4–6h prn. Migraine pain: 200–400 mg PO not to exceed 400 mg in 24 h unless directed by a physician (OTC dosing). Max dose 3.2 g/day.

PEDS — JRA: 30–50 mg/kg/day PO divided qGh. Max dose 2400 mg/24 h. 20 mg/kg/day may be adequate for milder disease. Analgesic/antipyretic, age older than 6 mo: 5–10 mg/kg PO q6–8h, prn. Max dose 40 mg/kg/day. Patent ductus arteriosus in neonates 32 weeks' gestational age or younger weighing 500–1500 g (NeoProfen): Specialized dosing.

FORMS — OTC: Caps/Liqui-Gel caps 200 mg. Tabs 100, 200 mg. Chewable tabs 100 mg. Susp (infant gtts) 50 mg/1.25 mL (with calibrated dropper), 100 mg/5 mL. Rx Generic/Trade: Tabs 400, 600, 800 mg.

NOTES — May antagonize antiplatelet effects of aspirin if given simultaneously. Take aspirin 2 h prior to ibuprofen. Administer IV (Caldolor) over at least 30 min; hydration important.

MOA — Anti-inflammatory/antipyretic, analgesic.

ADVERSE EFFECTS — Serious: Hypersensitivity, GI bleeding, nephrotoxicity. Frequent: Nausea, dyspepsia.

[7]**NAPROXEN** *(Naprosyn, Aleve, Anaprox, EC-Naprosyn, Naprelan, Prevacid, NapraPAC)*

▶L ✪ ♀B (D in 3rd trimester) ▶+ $ ■

WARNING — Multiple strengths; see FORMS and write specific product on Rx.

ADULT — RA/OA, ankylosing spondylitis, pain, dysmenorrhea, acute tendinitis and bursitis, fever: 250–500 mg PO two times per day. Delayed-release: 375–500 mg PO two times per day (do not crush or chew). Controlled-release: 750–1000 mg PO daily. Acute gout: 750 mg PO once, then 250 mg PO q8h until the attack subsides. Controlled-release: 1000–1500 mg PO once, then 1000 mg PO daily until the attack subsides.

PEDS — JRA: 10–20 mg/kg/day PO divided two times per day (up to 1250 mg/24 h). Pain for age older than 2 yo: 5–7 mg/kg/dose PO q8–12h.

UNAPPROVED ADULT — Acute migraine: 750 mg PO once, then 250–500 mg PO pm. Migraine prophylaxis, menstrual migraine: 500 mg PO two times per day beginning 1 day prior to onset of menses and ending on last day of period.

FORMS — OTC Generic/Trade (Aleve): Tabs, immediate-release 200 mg. OTC Trade only (Aleve): Caps, Gelcaps, immediate-release 200 mg. Rx Generic/Trade: Tabs, immediate-release (Naprosyn) 250, 375, 500 mg. (Anaprox) 275, 550 mg. Tabs, delayed-release enteric-coated (EC-Naprosyn) 375, 500 mg. Tabs, controlled-release (Naprelan) 375, 500, 750 mg. Susp (Naprosyn) 125 mg/5 mL. Prevacid NapraPAC: 7 lansoprazole 15 mg caps packaged with 14 naproxen tabs 375 mg or 500 mg.

NOTES — All dosing is based on naproxen content: 500 mg naproxen is equivalent to 550 mg naproxen sodium.

MOA — Anti-inflammatory, analgesic.
ADVERSE EFFECTS — Serious: Hypersensitivity, GI bleeding, nephrotoxicity. Frequent: Nausea, dyspepsia.

[8]DICLOFENAC (Voltaren, Voltaren XR, Flector, Zipsor, Cambia, Zorvolex, Voltaren Rapide)

▶L ⊗ ♀B (D in 3rd trimester) ▶+ $$$ ■

WARNING — Multiple strengths; see FORMS and write specific product on Rx.

ADULT — OA: Immediate- or delayed-release: 50 mg PO two to three times per day or 75 mg two times per day. Extended-release 100 mg PO daily. Gel: Apply 4 g to knees or 2 g to hands four times per day using enclosed dosing card. RA: Immediate- or delayed-release 50 mg PO three to four times per day or 75 mg two times per day. Extended-release 100 mg PO one to two times per day. Ankylosing spondylitis: Immediate- or delayed-release 25 mg PO four times per day and at bedtime. Analgesia and primary dysmenorrhea: Immediate- or delayed-release 50 mg PO three times per day. Acute pain in strains, sprains, or contusions: Apply 1 patch to painful area two times per day. Acute migraine with or without aura: 50 mg single dose (Cambia), mix packet with 30–60 mL water.

PEDS — Not approved in children.

UNAPPROVED PEDS — JRA: 2–3 mg/kg/day PO.

FORMS — Generic/Trade: Tabs, extended-release (Voltaren XR) 100 mg. Topical gel (Voltaren) 1% 100 g tube. Generic only: Tabs, immediate-release: 25, 50 mg. Generic only: Tabs, delayed-release: 25, 50, 75 mg. Trade only: Patch (Flector) 1.3% diclofenac epolamine. Trade only: Caps, liquid-filled (Zipsor) 25 mg. Caps (Zorvolex) 18, 35 mg. Trade only: Powder for oral soln (Cambia) 50 mg.

NOTES – Check LFTs at baseline, within 4–8 weeks of initiation, then periodically. Do not apply patch to damaged or nonintact skin. Wash hands, and avoid eye contact when handling the patch. Do not wear patch while bathing or showering.

MOA – Anti-inflammatory, analgesic.

ADVERSE EFFECTS – Serious: Hypersensitivity, GI bleeding, hepato/nephrotoxicity. Frequent: Nausea, dyspepsia, pruritus and dermatitis with patch and gel.

[9]KETOROLAC *(Toradol)*

▶L ⊗ ♀B (D in 3rd trimester) ▶– $$ ■

WARNING – Indicated for short-term (up to 5 days) therapy only. Ketorolac is a potent NSAID and can cause serious GI and renal adverse effects. It may also increase the risk of bleeding by inhibiting platelet function. Contraindicated in patients with active peptic ulcer disease, recent GI bleeding or perforation, a history of peptic ulcer disease or GI bleeding, or advanced renal impairment.

ADULT – Moderately severe, acute pain, single-dose treatment: 30–60 mg IM or 15–30 mg IV. Multiple-dose treatment: 15–30 mg IV/IM q6h. IV/IM doses are not to exceed 60 mg/day for age 65 yo or older, wt <50 kg, and patients with moderately elevated serum creatinine. Oral continuation therapy: 1.0 mg PO q4–6h prn, max dose 40 mg/day. Combined duration IV/IM and PO is not to exceed 5 days.

PEDS – Not approved in children.

UNAPPROVED PEDS – Pain: 0.5 mg/kg/dose IM/IV q6h (up to 30 mg q6h or 120 mg/day), give 10 mg PO q6h prn (up to 40 mg/day) for wt > 50 kg.

FORMS – Generic only: Tabs 10 mg.

MOA – Serious: Hypersensitivity, GI bleeding, nephrotoxicity. Frequent: Nausea, dyspepsia.

[10]DICLOFENAC—TOPICAL *(Solaraze, Voltaren, Pennsaid)*

▶L ♀C Category D at 30 weeks gestation and beyond. Avoid use starting at 30 weeks gestation. ▶? $$$ ■

WARNING – Risk of cardiovascular and GI events.

ADULT – Actinic/solar keratosis: Apply two times per day to lesions for 60–90 days (Solaraze). Osteoarthritis of areas amenable to topical therapy: 2 g (upper extremities) to 4 g (lower extremities) four times per day (Voltaren). 40 gtts to knee(s) four times daily.

PEDS – Not approved in children.

FORMS – Generic/Trade: Gel 3% (Solaraze) 100 g. Soln 1.5% (Pennsaid) 150 mL. Trade only: Gel 1% (Voltaren) 100 g. Soln 2.0% pump (pennsaid) 112 g.

NOTES – Avoid exposure to sun and sunlamps. Use caution in aspirin-sensitive patients. When using for OA (Voltaren), max daily dose 16 g to any single lower extremity joint, 8 g to any single upper extremity joint. Avoid use in setting of aspirin allergy or CABG surgery.

MOA – Inhibits prostaglandins at level of cyclooxygenase.

ADVERSE EFFECTS – Frequent: Rash, abdominal cramps, nausea, indigestion.

[11]LIDOCAINE-TOPICAL *(Xylocaine, Lidoderm, Numby Stuff, L-M-X, Zingo, Maxilene)*

▶LK ♀B ▶+ $

WARNING – Contraindicated in allergy to amide-type anesthetics.

ADULT – Topical anesthesia: Apply to affected area prn. Dose varies with anesthetic procedure, degree of anesthesia required, and individual patient response. Post-herpetic neuralgia (patch): Apply up to 3 patches to affected area at once for up to 12 h within a 24 h period.

PEDS – Topical anesthesia: Apply to affected area prn. Dose varies with anesthetic procedure, degree of anesthesia required, and individual patient response. Max 3 mg/kg/dose, do not repeat dose within 2 h. Intradermal powder injection for venipuncture/IV cannulation, for age 3–18 yo (Zingo): 0.5 mg to site 1–10 min prior.

UNAPPROVED PEDS – Topical anesthesia prior to venipuncture: Apply 30 min prior to procedure (ELA-Max 4%).

FORMS – For membranes of mouth and pharynx: Spray 10%, oint 5%, liquid 5%, soln 2%, 4% dental patch. For urethral use: Jelly 2%. Patch (Lidoderm $$$$$) 5%. Intradermal powder injection system: 0.5 mg (Zingo). OTC Trade only: Liposomal lidocaine 4% (ELA-Max).

NOTES – Apply patches only to intact skin to cover the most painful area. Patches may be cut into smaller sizes with scissors prior to removal of the release liner. Store and dispose out of the reach of children and pets to avoid possible toxicity from ingestion.

MOA – Anesthetic.

ADVERSE EFFECTS – Frequent: Skin irritation. Severe: CNS effects, bradycardia, bronchospasm, hypotension, allergic reactions.

[12]CAPSAICIN (Zostrix, Zostrix-HP, Qutenza)

▶? ♀? ▶? $

ADULT – Pain due to RA, OA, and neuralgias such as zoster or diabetic neuropathies: Apply to affected area up to three to four times per day. Post-herpetic neuralgia: 1 patch (Qutenza) applied for 1 hour in medical office, may repeat every 3 months.

PEDS — Children older than 2 yo: Pain due to RA, OA, and neuralgias such as zoster or diabetic neuropathies: Apply to affected area up to three to four times per day.

UNAPPROVED ADULT — Psoriasis and intractable pruritus, postmastectomy/postamputation neuromas (phantom limb pain), vulvar vestibulitis, apocrine chromhidrosis, and reflex sympathetic dystrophy.

FORMS — Rx: Patch 8% (Qutenza). OTC: Generic/Trade: Cream 0.025% 60 g, 0.075% (HP) 60 g. OTC Generic only: Lotion 0.025% 59 mL, 0.075% 59 mL.

NOTES — Burning occurs in 30% or more of patients but diminishes with continued use. Pain more commonly occurs when applied less than three to four times per day. Wash hands immediately after application.

MOA — Counter-irritant, releases substance P.

ADVERSE EFFECTS — Frequent: Burning, redness, sensation of warmth.

---

[13]**MORPHINE** *(MS Contin, Kadian, Avinza, Roxanol, Oramorph SR, MSIR, DepoDur, Statex, M.O.S. Doloral, M-Eslon)*

▶LK ✪ ♀C ▶+ ©II Varies by therapy ■

WARNING — Multiple strengths; see FORMS and write specific product on Rx. Drinking alcohol while taking Avinza may result in a rapid release of a potentially fatal dose of morphine.

ADULT — Moderate to severe pain: 10–30 mg PO q4h (immediate-release tabs, or oral soln). Controlled-release (MS Contin, Oramorph SR): 30 mg PO q8–12h. (Kadian): 20 mg PO q12–24h. Extended-release caps (Avinza): 30 mg PO daily. 10 mg q4h IM/SC. 2.5–15 mg/70 kg IV over 4–5 min. 10–20 mg

PR q4h. Pain with major surgery (DepoDur): 10–15 mg once epidurally at the lumbar level prior to surgery (max dose 20 mg), or 10 mg epidurally after clamping of the umbilical cord with cesarean section.

PEDS — Moderate to severe pain: 0.1–0.2 mg/kg up to 15 mg IM/SC/IV q2–4h.

UNAPPROVED PEDS — Moderate to severe pain: 0.2–0.5 mg/kg/dose PO (immediate-release) q4–6h. 0.3–0.6 mg/kg/dose PO (controlled-release) q12h.

FORMS — Generic only: Tabs, immediate-release 15, 30 mg ($). Oral soln 10 mg/5 mL, 20 mg/5 mL, 20 mg/mL (concentrate). Rectal supps 5, 10, 20, 30 mg. Generic/Trade: Controlled-release tabs (MS Contin) 15, 30, 60, 100, 200 mg ($$$$). Controlled-release caps (Kadian) 10, 20, 30, 50, 60, 80, 100 mg ($$$$$). Extended-release caps (Avinza) 30, 45, 60, 75, 90, 120 mg. Trade only: Controlled-release caps (Kadian) 40, 200 mg.

NOTES — Titrate dose as high as necessary to relieve cancer or nonmalignant pain where chronic opioids are necessary. The active metabolites may accumulate in hepatic/renal insufficiency and the elderly leading to increased analgesic and sedative effects. Do not break, chew, or crush MS Contin or Oramorph SR. Kadian and Avinza caps may be opened and sprinkled in applesauce for easier administration; however, the pellets should not be crushed or chewed. Doses more than 1600 mg/day of Avinza contain a potentially nephrotoxic quantity of fumaric acid. Do not mix DepoDur with other medications; do not administer any other medications into epidural space for at least 48 h. Severe opiate overdose with respiratory depression has occurred with intrathecal leakage of DepoDur.

MOA — Opioid agonist analgesic.

ADVERSE EFFECTS – Serious: Respiratory depression/arrest. Frequent: N/V, constipation, sedation, hypotension.

[14]FENTANYL (IONSYS, Duragesic, Actiq, Fentora, Sublimaze, Abstral, Subsys, Lazanda, Onsolis)

▶L ⊗ ♀C ▶+ ©II Varies by therapy

WARNING – Duragesic patches, Actiq, Fentora, Abstral, Subsys, and Lazanda are contraindicated in the management of acute or postop pain due to potentially life-threatening respiratory depression in opioid nontolerant patients. Instruct patients and their caregivers that even used patches/lozenges on a stick can be fatal to a child or pet. Dispose via toilet. Actiq and Fentora are not interchangeable. IONSYS: For hospital use only; remove prior to discharge. Can cause life-threatening respiratory depression.

ADULT – Duragesic patches: Chronic pain: 12–100 mcg/h patch q72h. Titrate dose to the needs of the patient. Some patients require q48h dosing. May wear more than 1 patch to achieve the correct analgesic effect. Actiq: Breakthrough cancer pain: 200–1600 mcg sucked over 15 min; if 200 mcg ineffective for 6 units use higher strength. Goal is 4 lozenges on a stick/day in conjunction with long-acting opioid. Buccal tab (Fentora) for breakthrough cancer pain: 100–800 mcg, titrated to pain relief; may repeat once after 30 min during single episode of breakthrough pain. See prescribing information for dose conversion from transmucosal lozenges. Buccal soluble film (Onsolis) for breakthrough cancer pain: 200–1200 mcg titrated to pain relief; no more than 4 doses/day separated by at least 2 h. Postop analgesia: 50–100 mcg IM; repeat in 1–2 h prn. SL tab (Abstral) for breakthrough cancer pain: 100 mcg, may repeat once after 30 min. Specialized titration. SL spray (Subsys) for breakthrough cancer pain 100 mcg, may repeat once after 30 min. Specialized titration. Nasal spray (Lazanda) for breakthrough cancer pain: 100 mcg. Specialized titration. IONSYS: Acute postop pain: Specialized dosing.

PEDS — Transdermal (Duragesic): Not approved in children younger than 2 yo or in opioid-naïve. Use adult dosing for age older than 2 yo. Children converting to a 25 mcg patch should be receiving 45 mg or more oral morphine equivalents/day. Actiq: Not approved for age younger than 16 yo. IONSYS not approved in children. Abstral, Subsys, and Lazanda: Not approved for age younger than 18 yo.

UNAPPROVED ADULT — Analgesia/procedural sedation/labor analgesia: 50–100 mcg IV or IM q1–2h prn.

UNAPPROVED PEDS — Analgesia: 1–2 mcg/kg/dose IV/IM q30–60 min prn or continuous IV infusion 1–3 mcg/kg/h (not to exceed adult dosing). Procedural sedation: 2–3 mcg/kg/dose for age 1–3 yo; 1–2 mcg/kg/dose for age 3–12 yo, 0.5–1 mcg/kg/dose (not to exceed adult dosing) for age older than 12 yo, procedural sedation doses may be repeated q30–60 min prn.

FORMS — Generic/Trade: Transdermal patches 12, 25, 50, 75, 100 mcg/h. Actiq lozenges on a stick, berry-flavored 200, 400, 600, 800, 1200, 1600 mcg. Trade only: (Fentora) buccal tab 100, 200, 400, 600, 800 mcg, packs of 4 or 28 tabs. Trade only: (Onsolis) buccal soluble film 200, 400, 600, 800, 1200 mcg in child-resistant, protective foil, packs of 30 films. Trade only: (Abstral) SL tabs 100, 200, 300, 400, 600, 800 mcg, packs of 4 or 32 tabs. Trade only: (Subsys) SL spray 100, 200, 400, 600, 800, 1200, 1600 mcg blister packs in cartons of 10 and

30 (30 only for 1200 and 1600 mcg). Trade only: (Lazanda) nasal spray 100, 400 mcg/spray, 8 sprays/bottle.

NOTES – Do not use patches for acute pain or in opioid-naïve patients. Oral transmucosal fentanyl doses of 5 mcg/kg provide effects similar to 0.75–1.25 mcg/kg of fentanyl IM. Lozenges on a stick should be sucked, not chewed. Flush lozenge remnants (without stick) down the toilet. For transdermal systems: Apply patch to non-hairy skin. Clip (do not shave) hair if you have to apply to hairy area. Fever or external heat sources may increase fentanyl released from patch. Patch should be removed prior to MRI and reapplied after the test. Dispose of a used patch by folding with the adhesive side of the patch adhering to itself then flush it down the toilet immediately. Do not cut the patch in half. For Duragesic patches and Actiq lozenges on a stick: Titrate dose as high as necessary to relieve cancer or nonmalignant pain where chronic opioids are necessary. Do not suck, chew, or swallow buccal tab. IONSYS: Apply to intact skin on the chest or upper arm. Each dose activated by the patient is delivered over a 10-min period. Remove prior to hospital discharge. Do not allow gel to touch mucous membranes. Dispose using gloves. Keep all forms of fentanyl out of the reach of children or pets. Concomitant use with potent CYP3A4 inhibitors such as ritonavir, ketoconazole, itraconazole, clarithromycin, nelfinavir, and nefazodone may result in an increase in fentanyl plasma concentrations, which could increase or prolong adverse drug effects and may cause potentially fatal respiratory depression. Onsolis is available only through the FOCUS Program and requires prescriber, pharmacy, and patient enrollment. Used films should be discarded into toilet. Abstral, Subsys, and Lazanda: Outpatients, prescribers, pharmacies, and distributors must be enrolled in TIRF REMS Access program before patient may receive medication.

MOA – Opioid agonist analgesic.

ADVERSE EFFECTS – Serious: Respiratory depression/arrest, chest wall rigidity. Frequent: N/V, constipation, sedation, skin irritation, dental decay with Actiq.

[15]HYDROMORPHONE *(Dilaudid, Exalgo, Hydromorph Contin)*

▶L ⊘ ♀C ▷? ⊙ll $$ ■

ADULT – Moderate to severe pain: 2–4 mg PO q4–6h. Initial dose (opioid-naïve): 0.5–2 mg SC/IM or slow IV q4–6h prn. 3 mg PR q6–8h. Controlled-release tabs: 8–64 mg daily.

PEDS – Not approved in children.

UNAPPROVED PEDS – Pain age 12 yo or younger: 0.03–0.08 mg/kg PO q4–6h prn. 0.015 mg/kg/dose IV q4–6h prn, use adult dose for older than 12 yo.

FORMS – Generic/Trade: Tabs 2, 4, 8 mg (8 mg trade scored). Oral soln 5 mg/5 mL. Controlled-release tabs (Exalgo): 8, 12, 16, 32 mg.

NOTES – In opioid-naïve patients, consider an initial dose of 0.5 mg or less IM/SC/IV. SC/IM/IV doses after initial dose should be individualized. May be given by slow IV injection over 2–5 min. Titrate dose as high as necessary to relieve cancer or nonmalignant pain where chronic opioids are necessary. 1.5 mg IV = 7.5 mg PO. Exalgo intended for opioid-tolerant patients only.

MOA – Opioid agonist analgesic.

ADVERSE EFFECTS – Serious: Respiratory depression/arrest. Frequent: N/V, constipation, sedation.

[16]SUFENTANIL *(Sufenta)*

▶L ♀C ▶? ©II $$

ADULT – General anesthesia: Induction: 8–30 mcg/kg IV; maintenance 0.5–10 mcg/kg IV. Conscious sedation: Loading dose: 0.1–0.5 mcg/kg; maintenance infusion 0.005–0.01 mcg/kg/min.

PEDS – General anesthesia: Induction: 8–30 mcg/kg IV; maintenance 0.5–10 mcg/kg IV. Conscious sedation: Loading dose: 0.1–0.5 mcg/kg; maintenance infusion 0.005–0.01 mcg/kg/min.

MOA – Serious: Respiratory depression, hypotension, bradycardia, chest wall rigidity, opiate dependence, hypersensitivity. Frequent: Sedation, N/V.

[17]NORCO *(hydrocodone + acetaminophen)*

▶L ✖ ♀C ▶? ©II $$

WARNING – Multiple strengths; see FORMS and write specific product on Rx.

ADULT – Moderate to severe pain: 1–2 tabs PO q4–6h prn (5/325), max dose 12 tabs/day. 1 tab (7.5/325 and 10/325) PO q4–6h prn, max dose 8 and 6 tabs/day, respectively.

PEDS – Not approved in children.

FORMS – Generic/Trade: Tabs 5/325, 7.5/325, 10/325 mg hydrocodone/acetaminophen, scored. Generic only: Soln 7.5/325 mg per 15 mL.

[18]VICODIN *(hydrocodone + acetaminophen)*

▶LK ✖ ♀C ▶? ©II $$$

WARNING – Multiple strengths; see FORMS and write specific product on Rx.

ADULT – Moderate pain: 5/300 mg (max dose 8 tabs/day) and 7.5/300 mg (max dose of 6 tabs/day): 1–2 tabs PO q4–6h prn. 10/300 mg: 1 tab PO q4–6h prn (max of 6 tabs/day).

PEDS – Not approved in children.

FORMS – Generic/Trade: Tabs Vicodin (5/300), Vicodin ES (7.5/300), Vicodin HP (10/300) mg hydrocodone/mg acetaminophen, scored.

[18]LORTAB *(hydrocodone + acetaminophen)*

▶LK ☒ ♀C ▶– ⊙II $$

WARNING – Multiple strengths; see FORMS and write specific product on Rx.

ADULT – Moderate pain: 1–2 tabs 2.5/325 and 5/325 PO q4–6h prn, max dose 8 tabs/day. 1 tab 7.5/325 and 10/325 PO q4–6h prn, max dose 5 tabs/day.

PEDS – Not approved in children.

FORMS – Generic/Trade: Lortab 5/325 (scored), Lortab 7.5/325 (trade scored), Lortab 10/325 mg hydrocodone/mg acetaminophen. Generic only: Tabs 2.5/325 mg.

MOA – Serious: Respiratory depression/arrest, hepatotoxicity. Frequent: N/V, constipation, sedation.

[18]LORCET *(hydrocodone + acetaminophen)*

▶LK ☒ ♀C ▶– ⊙II $$

WARNING – Multiple strengths; see FORMS and write specific product on Rx.

ADULT – Moderate pain: 1–2 caps (5/325) PO q4–6h prn, max dose 8 caps/day. 1 tab PO q4–6h prn (7.5/325 and 10/325), max dose 6 tabs/day.

PEDS – Not approved in children.
FORMS – Generic/Trade: Tabs, 5/325, 7.5/325,10/325 mg.

[19]VICOPROFEN *(hydrocodone + ibuprofen)*

▶LK ⊘ ♀– ▶? ©ΙΙ $$
ADULT – Moderate pain: 1 tab PO q4–6h prn, max dose 5 tabs/day.
PEDS – Not approved in children.
FORMS – Generic only: Tabs 2.5/200, 5/200,7.5/200, 10/200 mg hydrocodone/ibuprofen.
NOTES – See NSAIDs—Other subclass warning.
MOA – Combination analgesic.
ADVERSE EFFECTS – Serious: Respiratory depression/arrest, hypersensitivity, GI bleeding, nephrotoxicity. Frequent: N/V, constipation, dyspepsia, sedation.

[20]PERCOCET *(oxycodone + acetaminophen, Percocet-Demi, Oxycocet, Endocet)*

▶L ⊘ ♀C ▶ – ©ΙΙ $
WARNING – Multiple strengths; see FORMS and write specific product on Rx.
ADULT – Moderate to severe pain: 1–2 tabs PO q4–6h prn (2.5/325 and 5/325 mg). 1 tab PO q4–6h prn (7.5/325 and 10/325 mg).
PEDS – Not approved in children.
FORMS – Generic/Trade: Oxycodone/acetaminophen tabs 2.5/325, 5/325, 7.5/325, 10/325 mg. Trade only: (Prim lev) tabs 2.5/300, 5/300, 7.5/300, 10/300 mg. Generic only: 10/325 mg.

[20]ROXICET *(oxycodone + acetaminophen)*

▶L ⊗ ♀C ▶− ©II $

WARNING – Multiple strengths; see FORMS and write specific product on Rx.

ADULT – Moderate to severe pain: 1 tab PO q6h prn. Oral soln: 5 mL PO q6h prn.

PEDS – Not approved in children.

FORMS – Generic/Trade: Tabs 5/325 mg. Caps/caplets 5/325 mg. Soln 5/325 per 5 mL mg oxycodone/acetaminophen.

BACK PAIN (NON-RADICULAR)

Inpatient Analgesics (in the ED)	Outpatient Analgesics (discharge)
Non-Opioid	**Non-Opioid**
<u>Oral/Topical Analgesics:</u> [1]**Acetaminophen:** 500 mg, best if combined with NSAIDs [2]**Ibuprofen:** 400 mg, or [3]**Naproxen:** 500 mg, or [4]**Diclofenac:** 50 mg, or [5]**Ketorolac:** 10 mg [6]**Topical Diclofenac Gel/Patch:** a single patch to the affected area [7]**Topical Lidocaine** (4–5% patch, 2% cream): up to two patches to the affected area **Trigger point injection:** up to 10 mL 0.5% [8]**Bupivacaine,** or 10 mL of 1% [9]**Lidocaine** to site of maximal pain <u>Associated Muscle Spasm Only (not for routine use):</u> [10]**Methocarbamol:** 500–1500 mg in the ED (start at 250–500 mg per dose in elderly patients)	[2]**PO Ibuprofen:** 400 mg q8h × 3 days (max 5 days with 1200 mg/d) [1]**PO Acetaminophen:** 500 mg po q8h × 3 days (max 1500 mg/day). Best if combined with [2]**Ibuprofen** at 400 mg q8h or [3]**Naproxen** at 500 mg q12h [13]**PO Diflunisal** (Dolobid): 250–500 mg PO q12h × 3 days [3]**PO Naproxen:** 500 mg q12h × 3 days (max 5 days) [4]**PO Diclofenac:** 50 mg q8h × 3 days (max 5 days) [10]**PO Methocarbamol:** 500 mg q6–8h for 2–3 days, methocarbamol or cyclobenzaprine

(*continues*)

Inpatient Analgesics (in the ED)	Outpatient Analgesics (discharge)
Non-Opioid	**Non-Opioid**
[11]Cyclobenzaprine: 5–10 mg (start with 5 mg in elderly) **Parenteral Regimen:** [5]IV Ketorolac: 10–15 mg IVP (analgesic ceiling dose) [11]IV Lidocaine: 1.5 mg/kg of 2% (preservative-free lidocaine-cardiac or pre-made bags only) over 15 min (max dose 200 mg) [1]IV Acetaminophen: 1 g over 15 min (as adjunct to opioid/non-opioid) if patients are NPO/NPR or contraindications to opioids, NSAIDs, lidocaine, or ketamine [12]Ketamine (Subdissociative Dose, SDK) • **IV:** 0.3 mg/kg over 15 min, +/– continuous IV infusion at 0.15–0.2 mg/kg/h • **SQ** 0.3 mg/kg over 15 min, +/– continuous SQ infusion at 0.15–0.2 mg/kg/h	[11]Cyclobenzaprine: 5–10 mg (start with 5 mg in elderly). Only with proven muscle spasm. Not for routine treatment of back pain. [6]Topical Diclofenac Gel/Patch: Apply patch to affected area q12h for 5–7 days [7]Topical Lidocaine (4–5% patch, 2% cream): apply up to 2 patches to affected area for 12 h, then 12 h patch-free period [14]Topical Capsaicin (0.025–0.15% cream): apply q12h to affected area × 5–7 days. Avoid contact with mucous membranes **Physical Therapy**

(*continues*)

Inpatient Analgesics (in the ED)	Outpatient Analgesics (discharge)
• **Intranasal (IN):** 0.5–1 mg/kg (weight-based) q5–10 min (consider using highly concentrated solutions: Adults: 100 mg/mL, Peds: 50 mg/mL. No more than 0.3–0.5 mL/per nostril)	
Opioid	**Opioid**
Opioids (severe traumatic pain, intractable pain, failed non-opioid analgesia). Not to be used routinely in the ED. **Oral Regimen:** (for opioid-naïve patients) [15]**Morphine:** Morphine Sulfate Immediate Release (MSIR): 15 mg [16]**Fentanyl:** Transbuccal 100–200 µg dissolvable tablets; repeat at 60 min if pain persists [17]**Hydromorphone:** 2 mg **Parenteral Regimen:** [15]**Morphine:** • **IV:** 0.05–0.1 mg/kg (weight-based), titrate q10–20 min	Opioids (severe traumatic pain, intractable pain, failed non-opioid analgesia in opioid-naïve patients). Not to be used routinely in the ED. [15]**Morphine Sulfate Immediate Release (MSIR):** 15 mg q6–8h × 2–3 days (opioid-naïve patients) [19]**Hydrocodone/Acetaminophen (Norco)** 5/325 mg: 1–2 tabs q6–8h × 2–3 days [20]**Hydrocodone/Acetaminophen (Vicodin, Lortab, Lorcet)** 5/300 mg: 1–2 tabs q6–8h × 2–3 days

BACK PAIN (Non-Radicular)

(*continues*)

Inpatient Analgesics (in the ED)	Outpatient Analgesics (discharge)
Opioid	**Opioid**
• **IV:** 4–6 mg (fixed), titrate q10–20 min • **SQ:** 4–6 mg (fixed), re-administer as needed at q30–40 min • **IM:** 4–6 mg (fixed), re-administer as needed at q30–40 min (IM route should be avoided due to pain upon injection, muscle fibrosis, necrosis, increase in dosing requirements) **Nebulized** (via Breath Actuated Nebulizer [BAN]): Adults: 10–20 mg (fixed), repeat q15–20 min up to three doses Peds: 0.2–0.4 mg/kg (weight-based), repeat q15–20 min up to three doses • **PCA:** Demand dose: 1–2 mg Continuous basal infusion: 0.5–2 mg/h	[21]**Hydrocodone/Ibuprofen (Vicoprofen):** 5/200 mg: 1–2 tabs q6–8h × 2–3 days [22]**Oxycodone/Acetaminophen (Percocet, Roxicet):** 5/325 mg: 1–2 tabs q6–8h × 2–3 days [17]**Hydromorphone:** 2–4 mg q6–8h × 2–3 days (for opioid-naïve patients start with 2 mg dose)

(continues)

Inpatient Analgesics (in the ED)	Outpatient Analgesics (discharge)
Opioid	**Opioid**

[16]**Fentanyl:**
 	
• **IV:** 0.25–0.5 µg/kg (weight-based), titrate q10 min
• **IV:** 25–50 µg (fixed), titrate q10 min
  Nebulized (via BAN):
  Adults: 2–4 mg/kg (weight-based), titrate q20–30 min, up to three doses
  Peds: 2–4 mg/kg (weight-based), titrate q20–30 min, up to three doses
• **Intranasal (IN):** 1–2 µg/kg (weight-based), titrate q5–10 min (consider using highly concentrated solutions:
  Adults: 100 µg/mL
  Peds: 50 µg/mL. (No more than 0.3–0.5 mL/per nostril)
• **Transmucosal:** 15–20 mcg/kg lollipops
• **PCA:**
  Demand dose: 20–50 µg
  Continuous basal infusion: 0.05-0.1 µg/kg/h	

(*continues*)

Inpatient Analgesics (in the ED)	Outpatient Analgesics (discharge)
Opioid	**Opioid**
[17]Hydromorphone: • **IV:** 0.2–0.5 mg initial, titrate q10–15 min • **SQ:** 0.5–1 mg, titrate q30–40 min • **IM:** 0.5–1 mg, titrate q30–40 min (IM route should be avoided due to pain, muscle fibrosis, necrosis, increase in dosing requirements) • **PCA:** Demand dose: 0.2–0.4 mg Continuous basal infusion: 0.1–0.4 mg/h [18]Sufentanil: • **Intranasal (IN):** 0.5 µg/kg, titration q10 min up to three doses	

[1]**ACETAMINOPHEN** *(Tylenol, Panadol, Tempra, Ofirmev, Paracetamol, Abenol, Atasol, Pediatrix)*

▶LK ♀B ▶+$

ADULT – Analgesic/antipyretic: 325–1000 mg PO q4–6h pm. 650 mg PR q4–6h pm. Max dose 4 g/day. OA: Extended-release: 2 caps PO q8h around the clock. Max dose 6 caps/day.

PEDS – Analgesic/antipyretic: 10–15 mg/kg q4–6h PO/PR pm. Max 5 doses/day.

UNAPPROVED ADULT – OA: 1000 mg PO four times per day.

FORMS – OTC: Tabs 325, 500, 650 mg. Chewable tabs 80 mg. Orally disintegrating tabs 80, 160 mg. Caps/gelcaps 500 mg. Extended-release caplets 650 mg. Liquid 160 mg/5 mL, 500 mg/15 mL. Supps 80, 120, 325, 650 mg.

[2]**IBUPROFEN (Motrin, Advil, Nuprin, Rufen, NeoProfen, Caldolor)**

▶L ⊗ ♀B (D in 3rd trimester) ▶+ ■

ADULT – RA/OA, gout: 200–800 mg PO three to four times per day. Mild to moderate pain: 400 mg PO q4–6h. 400–800 mg IV (Caldolor) q6h prn. 400 mg IV (Caldolor) q4–6h or 100–200 mg q4h prn. Primary dysmenorrhea: 400 mg PO q4h prn. Fever: 200 mg PO q4–6h prn. Migraine pain: 200–400 mg PO not to exceed 400 mg in 24 h unless directed by a physician (OTC dosing). Max dose 3.2 g/day.

PEDS – JRA: 30–50 mg/kg/day PO divided qG h. Max dose 2400 mg/24 h. 20 mg/kg/day may be adequate for milder disease. Analgesic/antipyretic, age older than 6 mo: 5–10 mg/kg PO q6–8h prn. Max dose 40 mg/kg/day. Patent ductus arteriosus in neonates 32 weeks' gestational age or younger weighing 500–1500 g (NeoProfen): Specialized dosing.

FORMS – OTC: Caps/Liqui-Gel caps 200 mg. Tabs 100, 200 mg. Chewable tabs 100 mg. Susp (infant gtts) 50 mg/1.25 mL (with calibrated dropper), 100 mg/5 mL. Rx Generic/Trade: Tabs 400, 600, 800 mg.

NOTES – May antagonize antiplatelet effects of aspirin if given simultaneously. Take aspirin 2 h prior to ibuprofen. Administer IV (Caldolor) over at least 30 min; hydration important.
MOA – Anti-inflammatory/antipyretic, analgesic.
ADVERSE EFFECTS – Serious: Hypersensitivity, GI bleeding, nephrotoxicity. Frequent: Nausea, dyspepsia.

---

[3]NAPROXEN *(Naprosyn, Aleve, Anaprox, EC-Naprosyn, Naprelan, Prevacid, NapraPAC)*

▶L ⊘ ♀B (D in 3rd trimester) ▶+ ■
WARNING – Multiple strengths; see FORMS and write specific product on Rx.
ADULT – RA/OA, ankylosing spondylitis, pain, dysmenorrhea, acute tendinitis and bursitis, fever: 250–500 mg PO two times per day. Delayed-release: 375–500 mg PO two times per day (do not crush or chew). Controlled-release: 750–1000 mg PO daily. Acute gout: 750 mg PO once, then 250 mg PO q8h until the attack subsides. Controlled-release: 1000–1500 mg PO once, then 1000 mg PO daily until the attack subsides.
PEDS – JRA: 10–20 mg/kg/day PO divided two times per day (up to 1250 mg/24 h). Pain for age older than 2 yo: 5–7 mg/kg/dose PO q8–12h.
UNAPPROVED ADULT – Acute migraine: 750 mg PO once, then 250–500 mg PO prn. Migraine prophylaxis, menstrual migraine: 500 mg PO two times per day beginning 1 day prior to onset of menses and ending on last day of period.
FORMS – OTC Generic/Trade (Aleve): Tabs, immediate-release 200 mg. OTC Trade only (Aleve): Caps, Gelcaps, immediate-release 200 mg. Rx Generic/Trade: Tabs, immediate-release (Naprosyn) 250, 375, 500 mg. (Anaprox) 275, 550 mg. Tabs,

delayed-release enteric-coated (EC-Naprosyn) 375, 500 mg. Tabs, controlled-release (Naprelan) 375, 500, 750 mg. Susp (Naprosyn) 125 mg/5 mL. Prevacid NapraPAC: 7 lansoprazole 15 mg caps packaged with 14 naproxen tabs 375 mg or 500 mg.

NOTES – All dosing is based on naproxen content: 500 mg naproxen is equivalent to 550 mg naproxen sodium.

MOA – Anti-inflammatory, analgesic.

ADVERSE EFFECTS – Serious: Hypersensitivity, GI bleeding, nephrotoxicity. Frequent: Nausea, dyspepsia.

[4]DICLOFENAC *(Voltaren, Voltaren XR, Flector, Zipsor, Cambia, Zorvolex, Voltaren Rapide)*

▶L ⊗ ♀B (D in 3rd trimester) ▶ – $$$■

WARNING – Multiple strengths; see FORMS and write specific product on Rx.

ADULT – OA: Immediate- or delayed-release: 50 mg PO two to three times per day or 75 mg two times per day. Extended-release 100 mg PO daily. Gel: Apply 4 g to knees or 2 g to hands four times per day using enclosed dosing card. RA: Immediate- or delayed-release 50 mg PO three to four times per day or 75 mg two times per day. Extended-release 100 mg PO one to two times per day. Ankylosing spondylitis: Immediate- or delayed-release 25 mg PO four times per day and at bedtime. Analgesia and primary dysmenorrhea: Immediate- or delayed-release 50 mg PO three times per day. Acute pain in strains, sprains, or contusions: Apply 1 patch to painful area two times per day. Acute migraine with or without aura: 50 mg single dose (Cambia), mix packet with 30–60 mL water.

PEDS – Not approved in children.

UNAPPROVED PEDS – JRA: 2–3 mg/kg/day PO.

FORMS – Generic/Trade: Tabs, extended-release (Voltaren XR) 100 mg. Topical gel (Voltaren) 1% 100 g tube. Generic only: Tabs, immediate-release: 25, 50 mg. Generic only: Tabs, delayed-release: 25, 50, 75 mg. Trade only: Patch (Flector) 1.3% diclofenac epolamine. Trade only: Caps, liquid-filled (Zipsor) 25 mg. Caps (Zorvolex) 18, 35 mg. Trade only: Powder for oral soln (Cambia) 50 mg.

NOTES – Check LFTs at baseline, within 4–8 weeks of initiation, then periodically. Do not apply patch to damaged or nonintact skin. Wash hands, and avoid eye contact when handling the patch. Do not wear patch while bathing or showering.

MOA – Anti-inflammatory, analgesic.

ADVERSE EFFECTS – Serious: Hypersensitivity, GI bleeding, hepato/nephrotoxicity. Frequent: Nausea, dyspepsia, pruritus, and dermatitis with patch and gel.

[5]KETOROLAC *(Toradol)*

▶L ⊗ ♀B (D in 3rd trimester) ▶ + $■

WARNING – Indicated for short-term (up to 5 days) therapy only. Ketorolac is a potent NSAID and can cause serious GI and renal adverse effects. It may also increase the risk of bleeding by inhibiting platelet function. Contraindicated in patients with active peptic ulcer disease, recent GI bleeding or perforation, a history of peptic ulcer disease or GI bleeding, or advanced renal impairment.

ADULT – Moderately severe, acute pain, single-dose treatment: 30–60 mg IM or 15–30 mg IV. Multiple-dose treatment: 15–30 mg IV/IM q6h. IV/IM doses are not to exceed 60 mg/day for age 65 yo or older, wt < 50 kg, and patients with moderately elevated serum creatinine. Oral continuation therapy: 1.0 mg PO q4–6h prn, max dose 40 mg/day. Combined duration IV/IM and PO is not to exceed 5 days.

PEDS – Not approved in children.

UNAPPROVED PEDS – Pain: 0.5 mg/kg/dose IM/IV q6h (up to 30 mg q6h or 120 mg/day), give 10 mg PO qGh pm (up to 40 mg/day) for wt > 50 kg.

FORMS – Generic only: Tabs 10 mg.

MOA – Serious: Hypersensitivity, GI bleeding, nephrotoxicity. Frequent: Nausea, dyspepsia.

[6]DICLOFENAC-TOPICAL *(Solaraze, Voltaren, Pennsaid)*

▶? $$$ ■

WARNING – Risk of cardiovascular and GI events.

ADULT – Osteoarthritis of areas amenable to topical therapy: 2 g (upper extremities) to 4 g (lower extremities) four times per day (Voltaren). 40 gtts to knee(s) four times daily.

PEDS – Not approved in children.

FORMS – Generic/Trade: Gel 3% (Solaraze) 100 g. Soln 1.5% (Pennsaid) 150 mL. Trade only: Gel 1% (Voltaren) 100 g. Soln 2.0% Pump (Pennsaid) 112 g.

NOTES – Avoid exposure to sun and sunlamps. Use caution in aspirin-sensitive patients. When using for OA (Voltaren), max daily dose 16 g to any single lower extremity joint, 8 g to any single upper extremity joint. Avoid use in setting of aspirin allergy or CABG surgery.

MOA – Inhibits prostaglandins at level of cyclooxygenase.

ADVERSE EFFECTS – Frequent: Rash, abdominal cramps, nausea, indigestion.

[7]LIDOCAINE—TOPICAL *(Xylocaine, Lidoderm, Numby Stuff, LMX, Zingo, Maxilene)*

▶LK ♀C ▶+ $

WARNING — Contraindicated in allergy to amide-type anesthetics.

ADULT — Topical anesthesia: Apply to affected area prn. Dose varies with anesthetic procedure, degree of anesthesia required, and individual patient response. Postherpetic neuralgia (patch): Apply up to 3 patches to affected area at once for up to 12 h within a 24 h period.

PEDS — Topical anesthesia: Apply to affected area prn. Dose varies with anesthetic procedure, degree of anesthesia required, and individual patient response. Max 3 mg/kg/dose, do not repeat dose within 2 h. Intradermal powder injection for venipuncture/IV cannulation, for age 3 to 18 yo (Zingo): 0.5 mg to site 1–10 min prior.

UNAPPROVED PEDS — Topical anesthesia prior to venipuncture: Apply 30 min prior to procedure (ELA-Max 4%).

FORMS — For membranes of mouth and pharynx: Spray 10%, oint 5%, liquid 5%, soln 2%, 4% dental patch. For urethral use: Jelly 2%. Patch (Lidoderm $$$$$) 5%. Intradermal powder injection system: 0.5 mg (Zingo). OTC Trade only: Liposomal lidocaine 4% (ELA-Max).

NOTES — Apply patches only to intact skin to cover the most painful area. Patches may be cut into smaller sizes with scissors prior to removal of the release liner. Store and dispose out of the reach of children and pets to avoid possible toxicity from ingestion.

MOA — Anesthetic.

ADVERSE EFFECTS — Frequent: Skin irritation. Severe: CNS effects, bradycardia, bronchospasm, hypotension, allergic reactions.

[8]BUPIVACAINE *(Marcaine, Sensorcaine)*

▶LK ♀B ▶?$

ADULT — Local anesthesia, nerve block: 0.25% injection. Up to 2.5 mg/kg without epinephrine and up 3.0 mg/kg with epinephrine.

PEDS — Not recommended in children younger than 12 yo.

FORMS — 0.25%, 0.5%, 0.75%, all with or without epinephrine.

NOTES — Onset 5 min, duration 2–4 h (longer with epi). Amide group.

MOA — Amide local anesthetic.

ADVERSE EFFECTS — Serious: Seizures, cardiovascular depression, bradycardia, hypersensitivity, methemoglobinemia. Frequent: None.

[9]LIDOCAINE—LOCAL ANESTHETIC *(Xylocaine)*

▶LK ♀C ▶? $

ADULT — Without epinephrine: Max dose 4.5 mg/kg not to exceed 300 mg. With epinephrine: Max dose 7 mg/kg not to exceed 500 mg. Dose for regional block varies by region.

PEDS — Same as adult.

FORMS — 0.5, 1, 1.5, 2%. With epi: 0.5, 1, 1.5, 2%.

NOTES — Onset within 2 min, duration 30–60 min (longer with epi). Amide group. Use "cardiac lidocaine" (ie, IV formulation) for Bier blocks at max dose of 3 mg/kg so that neither epinephrine nor methylparaben are injected IV.

MOA — Amide local anesthetic.

ADVERSE EFFECTS — Serious: Seizures, cardiovascular depression, bradycardia, hypersensitivity, methemoglobinemia. Frequent: None.

[10]METHOCARBAMOL *(Robaxin, Robaxin-750)*

▶LK ♀C ▶? $

ADULT — Musculoskeletal pain, acute relief: 1500 mg PO four times per day or 1000 mg IM/IV three times per day for 48–72 h. Maintenance: 1000 mg PO four times per day, 750 mg PO q4 h, or 1500 mg PO three times per day. Tetanus: Specialized dosing.

PEDS — Tetanus: Specialized dosing.

FORMS — Generic/Trade: Tabs 500, 750 mg. OTC in Canada.

NOTES — Max IV rate of undiluted drug 3 mL/min to avoid syncope, hypotension, and bradycardia. Total parenteral dosage should not exceed 3 g/day for more than 3 consecutive days, except in the treatment of tetanus. Urine may turn brown, black, or green.

MOA — Skeletal muscle relaxant.

ADVERSE EFFECTS — Serious: Syncope, hypotension. Frequent: Drowsiness, dizziness, discolored urine (brown, black, green).

[11]CYCLOBENZAPRINE *(Amrix, Flexeril, Fexmid)*

▶LK ♀B ▶? $

ADULT — Musculoskeletal pain: 5–10 mg PO three times per day up to max dose of 30 mg/day or 15–30 mg (extended-release) PO daily. Not recommended in elderly or for use longer than 2–3 weeks.

PEDS — Not approved in children.

FORMS — Generic/Trade: Tabs 5, 7.5, 10 mg. Extended-release caps 15, 30 mg ($$$$$).

NOTES – Contraindicated with recent or concomitant MAOI use, immediately post ML, in patients with arrhythmias, conduction disturbances, heart failure, and hyperthyroidism. Not effective for cerebral or spinal cord disease or in children with cerebral palsy. May have similar adverse effects and drug interactions to TCAs. Caution with urinary retention, angle-closure glaucoma, increased intraocular pressure.

MOA – Skeletal muscle relaxant.

ADVERSE EFFECTS – Serious: Arrhythmia. Frequent: Drowsiness, dizziness, dry mouth, blurred vision.

[12]KETAMINE *(Ketalar)*

▶L ♀C ▶? ©III $■

WARNING – Post-anesthetic emergence reactions up to 24 h later manifested as dreamlike state, vivid imagery, hallucinations, and delirium reported in about 12% of cases. Incidence reduced when (1) age less than 15 yo or greater than 65 yo, (2) concomitant use of benzodiazepines, lower dose, or used as induction agent only (because of use of post-intubation sedation).

ADULT – Induction of anesthesia: Adult: 1–2 mg/kg IV over 1–2 min (produces 5–10 min dissociative state) or 6.5–13 mg/kg IM (produces 10–20 min dissociative state).

PEDS – Age over 16 yo: same as adult.

UNAPPROVED ADULT – Dissociative sedation: 1–2 mg/kg IV over 1–2 mm (sedation lasting 10–20 min); repeat 0.5 mg/kg doses every 5–15 min may be given; 4–5 mg/kg IM (sedation lasting 15–30 min); repeat 2–4 mg/kg IM can be given if needed after 10–15 min. Analgesia adjunct subdissociative dose: 0.01–0.5 mg/kg in conjunction with opioid analgesia.

UNAPPROVED PEDS – Dissociative sedation: Age older than 3 mo: 1–2 mg/kg IV (produces 5–10 min dissociative state) over 1–2 min or 4–5 mg/kg IM (produces 10–20 min dissociative state). Not approved for age younger than 3 mo.

FORMS – Generic/Trade: 10, 50, 100 mg/mL.

NOTES – Recent evidence suggests ketamine is not contraindicated in patients with head injuries. However, avoid if CAD or severe HTN. Concurrent administration of atropine no longer recommended. Consider prophylactic ondansetron to reduce vomiting and prophylactic midazolam (0.3 mg/kg) to reduce recovery reactions.

MOA – NMDA receptor antagonist which produces dissociative state.

ADVERSE EFFECTS – Serious: Laryngospasm, hallucinatory emergence reactions, hypersalivation. Frequent: Nystagmus, hypertension, tachycardia, N/V, muscular hypertonicity, myoclonus.

[13]DIFLUNISAL *(Dolobid)*

▶K ⊗ ♀C (D in 3rd trimester) ▶– $$$$■

ADULT – Mild to moderate pain: Initially, 500 mg to 1 g PO, then 250–500 mg PO q8–12 h. RA/OA: 500 mg to 1 g PO divided two times per day. Max dose 1.5 g/day.

PEDS – Not approved in children.

FORMS – Generic only: Tabs 500 mg.

NOTES – Do not crush or chew tabs; increases acetaminophen levels.

MOA – Anti-inflammatory, analgesic.

ADVERSE EFFECTS – Serious: Hypersensitivity, Reye's syndrome, GI bleeding, nephrotoxicity. Frequent: Nausea, dyspepsia.

[14]CAPSAICIN *(Zostrix, Zostrix-HP, Qutenza)*

▶? ♀? ▶? $

ADULT — Pain due to RA, OA, and neuralgias such as zoster or diabetic neuropathies: Apply to affected area up to three to four times per day. Post-herpetic neuralgia: 1 patch (Qutenza) applied for 1 h in medical office, may repeat every 3 months.

PEDS — Children older than 2 yo: Pain due to RA, OA, and neuralgias such as zoster or diabetic neuropathies: Apply to affected area up to three to four times per day.

UNAPPROVED ADULT — Psoriasis and intractable pruritus, post-mastectomy/post-amputation neuromas (phantom limb pain), vulvar vestibulitis, apocrine chromhidrosis, and reflex sympathetic dystrophy.

FORMS — Rx: Patch 8% (Qutenza). OTC: Generic/Trade: Cream 0.025% 60 g, 0.075% (HP) 60 g. OTC Generic only: Lotion 0.025% 59 mL, 0.075% 59 mL.

NOTES — Burning occurs in 30% or more of patients but diminishes with continued use. Pain more commonly occurs when applied less than three to four times per day. Wash hands immediately after application.

MOA — Counter-irritant, releases substance P.

ADVERSE EFFECTS — Frequent: Burning, redness, sensation of warmth.

[15]MORPHINE *(MS Contin, Kadian, Avinza, Roxanol, Oramorph SR, MSIR, DepoDur, Statex, M.O.S. Doloral, M-Eslon)*

▶K ⊗ ♀C (D in 3rd trimester) ▶+ $$$$■

WARNING – Multiple strengths; see FORMS and write specific product on Rx. Drinking alcohol while taking Avinza may result in a rapid release of a potentially fatal dose of morphine.

ADULT – Moderate to severe pain: 10–30 mg PO q4h (immediate-release tabs, or oral soln). Controlled-release (MS Contin, Oramorph SR): 30 mg PO q8–12h. (Kadian): 20 mg PO q12–24h. Extended-release caps (Avinza): 30 mg PO daily. 10 mg q4h IM/SC. 2.5–15 mg/70 kg IV over 4–5 min. 10–20 mg PR q4h. Pain with major surgery (DepoDur): 10–15 mg once epidurally at the lumbar level prior to surgery (max dose 20 mg), or 10 mg epidurally after clamping of the umbilical cord with cesarean section.

PEDS – Moderate to severe pain: 0.1–0.2 mg/kg up to 15 mg IM/SC/IV q2–4 h.

UNAPPROVED PEDS – Moderate to severe pain: 0.2–0.5 mg/kg/dose PO (immediate-release) q4–6h. 0.3–0.6 mg/kg/dose PO (controlled-release) q12h.

FORMS – Generic only: Tabs, immediate-release 15, 30 mg ($). Oral soln 10 mg/5 mL, 20 mg/5 mL, 20 mg/mL (concentrate). Rectal supps 5, 10, 20, 30 mg. Generic/Trade: Controlled-release tabs (MS Contin) 15, 30, 60, 100, 200 mg ($$$$). Controlled-release caps (Kadian) 10, 20, 30, 50, 60, 80, 100 mg ($$$$$). Extended-release caps (Avinza) 30, 45, 60, 75, 90, 120 mg. Trade only: Controlled-release caps (Kadian) 40, 200 mg.

NOTES – Titrate dose as high as necessary to relieve cancer or non-malignant pain where chronic opioids are necessary. The active metabolites may accumulate in hepatic/renal insufficiency and the elderly leading to increased analgesic and sedative effects. Do not break, chew, or crush MS Contin or Oramorph SR. Kadian and Avinza caps may be opened and sprinkled in applesauce for easier administration; however, the pellets should not be crushed or chewed. Doses more than 1600 mg/day of Avinza contain a potentially nephrotoxic quantity of fumaric acid. Do not mix DepoDur with other medications; do not administer any other medications into epidural space for at least 48 h. Severe opiate overdose with respiratory depression has occurred with intrathecal leakage of DepoDur.

MOA – Opioid agonist analgesic.

ADVERSE EFFECTS – Serious: Respiratory depression/arrest. Frequent: N/V, constipation, sedation, hypotension.

[16]FENTANYL (IONSYS, Duragesic, Actiq, Fentora, Sublimaze, Abstral, Subsys, Lazanda, Onsolis)

▶L ⊗ ♀C ▶+ ©II Varies by therapy ■

WARNING – Duragesic patches, Actiq, Fentora, Abstral, Subsys, and Lazanda are contraindicated in the management of acute or postop pain due to potentially life-threatening respiratory depression in opioid nontolerant patients. Instruct patients and their caregivers that even used patches/lozenges on a stick can be fatal to a child or pet. Dispose via toilet. Actiq and Fentora are not interchangeable. IONSYS: For hospital use only; remove prior to discharge. Can cause life-threatening respiratory depression.

ADULT – Duragesic patches: Chronic pain: 12–100 mcg/h patch q72h. Titrate dose to the needs of the patient. Some patients require q48h dosing. May wear more than 1 patch to achieve the correct analgesic effect. Actiq: Breakthrough cancer pain: 200–1600 mcg sucked over 15 min if 200 mcg ineffective for 6 units use higher strength. Goal is 4 lozenges

on a stick/day in conjunction with long-acting opioid. Buccal tab (Fentora) for breakthrough cancer pain: 100–800 mcg, titrated to pain relief; may repeat once after 30 min during single episode of breakthrough pain. See prescribing information for dose conversion from transmucosal lozenges. Buccal soluble film (Onsolis) for breakthrough cancer pain: 200–1200 mcg titrated to pain relief; no more than 4 doses/day separated by at least 2 h. Postop analgesia: 50–100 mcg IM; repeat in 1–2 h prn. SL tab (Abstral) for breakthrough cancer pain: 100 mcg, may repeat once after 30 min. Specialized titration. SL spray (Subsys) for breakthrough cancer pain 100 mcg, may repeat once after 30 min. Specialized titration. Nasal spray (Lazanda) for breakthrough cancer pain: 100 mcg. Specialized titration. IONSYS: Acute postop pain: Specialized dosing.
PEDS – Transdermal (Duragesic): Not approved in children younger than 2 yo or in opioid-naïve. Use adult dosing for age older than 2 yo. Children converting to a 25-mcg patch should be receiving 45 mg or more oral morphine equivalents/day. Actiq: Not approved for age younger than 16 yo. IONSYS not approved in children. Abstral, Subsys, and Lazanda: Not approved for age younger than 18 yo.
UNAPPROVED ADULT – Analgesia/procedural sedation/labor analgesia: 50–100 mcg IV or IM q1–2h prn.
UNAPPROVED PEDS – Analgesia: 1–2 mcg/kg/dose IV/IM q30–60 min prn or continuous IV infusion 1–3 mcg/kg/h (not to exceed adult dosing). Procedural sedation: 2–3 mcg/kg/dose for age 1–3 yo; 1–2 mcg/kg/dose for age 3–12 yo, 0.5–1 mcg/kg/dose (not to exceed adult dosing) for age older than 12 yo, procedural sedation doses may be repeated q30–60 min prn.

FORMS – Generic/Trade: Transdermal patches 12, 25, 50, 75, 100 mcg/h. Actiq lozenges on a stick, berry-flavored 200, 400, 600, 800, 1200, 1600 mcg. Trade only: (Fentora) buccal tab 100, 200, 400, 600, 800 mcg, packs of 4 or 28 tabs. Trade only: (Onsolis) buccal soluble film 200, 400, 600, 800, 1200 mcg in child-resistant, protective foil, packs of 30 films. Trade only: (Abstral) SL tabs 100, 200, 300, 400, 600, 800 mcg, packs of 4 or 32 tabs. Trade only: (Subsys) SL spray 100, 200, 400, 600, 800, 1200, 1600 mcg blister packs in cartons of 10 and 30 (30 only for 1200 and 1600 mcg). Trade only: (Lazanda) nasal spray 100, 400 mcg/spray, 8 sprays/bottle.

NOTES – Do not use patches for acute pain or in opioid-naïve patients. Oral transmucosal fentanyl doses of 5 mcg/kg provide effects similar to 0.75–1.25 mcg/kg of fentanyl IM. Lozenges on a stick should be sucked, not chewed. Flush lozenge remnants (without stick) down the toilet. For transdermal systems: Apply patch to non-hairy skin. Clip (do not shave) hair if you have to apply to hairy area. Fever or external heat sources may increase fentanyl released from patch. Patch should be removed prior to MRI and reapplied after the test. Dispose of a used patch by folding with the adhesive side of the patch adhering to itself then flush it down the toilet immediately. Do not cut the patch in half. For Duragesic patches and Actiq lozenges on a stick: Titrate dose as high as necessary to relieve cancer or nonmalignant pain where chronic opioids are necessary. Do not suck, chew, or swallow buccal tab. IONSYS: Apply to intact skin on the chest or upper arm. Each dose activated by the patient is delivered over a 10-min period. Remove prior to hospital discharge. Do not allow gel to touch mucous membranes. Dispose using gloves. Keep all forms of fentanyl out of the reach of children or pets. Concomitant use with potent CYP3A4 inhibitors such as ritonavir, ketoconazole, itraconazole, clarithromycin, nelfinavir, and nefazodone may result in an increase in fentanyl plasma concentrations, which could increase or prolong adverse drug effects and may cause potentially fatal respiratory depression. Onsolis is available only through the FOCUS Program and requires prescriber, pharmacy, and patient enrollment. Used films should be discarded into toilet. Abstral, Subsys, and Lazanda: Outpatients, prescribers, pharmacies, and distributors must be enrolled in TIRF REMS Access program before patient may receive medication.

MOA – Opioid agonist analgesic.

ADVERSE EFFECTS – Serious: Respiratory depression/arrest, chest wall rigidity. Frequent: N/V, constipation, sedation, skin irritation, dental decay with Actiq.

[17] HYDROMORPHONE *(Dilaudid, Exalgo, Hydromorph Contin)*

▶L ♀C ▶? ©II $$ ■

ADULT – Moderate to severe pain: 2–4 mg PO q4–6h. Initial dose (opioid-naïve): 0.5–2 mg SC/IM or slow IV q4–6h prn. 3 mg PR q6–8h. Controlled-release tabs: 8–64 mg daily.

PEDS – Not approved in children.

UNAPPROVED PEDS – Pain age 12 yo or younger: 0.03 to 0.08 mg/kg PO q4–6h prn. 0.015 mg/kg/dose IV q4–6h prn, use adult dose for older than 12 yo.

FORMS – Generic/Trade: Tabs 2, 4, 8 mg (8 mg trade scored). Oral soln 5 mg/5 mL. Controlled-release tabs (Exalgo): 8, 12, 16, 32 mg.

NOTES – In opioid-naïve patients, consider an initial dose of 0.5 mg or less IM/SC/IV. SC/IM/IV doses after initial dose should be individualized. May be given by slow IV injection over 2–5 min. Titrate dose as high as necessary to relieve cancer or nonmalignant pain where chronic opioids are necessary. 1.5 mg IV = 7.5 mg PO. Exalgo intended for opioid-tolerant patients only.

MOA – Opioid agonist analgesic.

ADVERSE EFFECTS – Serious: Respiratory depression/arrest. Frequent: N/V, constipation, sedation.

[18]SUFENTANIL *(Sufenta)*

▶L ♀C ▷? ©II $$

ADULT – General anesthesia: Induction: 8–30 mcg/kg IV; maintenance 0.5–10 mcg/kg IV. Conscious sedation: Loading dose: 0.1–0.5 mcg/kg; maintenance infusion 0.005–0.01 mcg/kg/min.

PEDS – General anesthesia: Induction: 8–30 mcg/kg IV; maintenance 0.5–10 mcg/kg IV. Conscious sedation: Loading dose: 0.1–0.5 mcg/kg; maintenance infusion 0.005–0.01 mcg/kg/min.

MOA – Serious: Respiratory depression, hypotension, bradycardia, chest wall rigidity, opiate dependence, hypersensitivity. Frequent: Sedation, N/V.

[19]NORCO *(hydrocodone + acetaminophen)*

▶L ⊗ ♀C ▷? ©II $$

WARNING – Multiple strengths; see FORMS and write specific product on Rx.

ADULT – Moderate to severe pain: 1–2 tabs PO q4–6h prn (5/325), max dose 12 tabs/day. 1 tab (7.5/325 and 10/325) PO q4–6h prn, max dose 8 and 6 tabs/day, respectively.
PEDS – Not approved in children.
FORMS – Generic/Trade: Tabs 5/325, 7.5/325, 10/325 mg hydrocodone/acetaminophen, scored. Generic only: Soln 7.5/325 mg per 15 mL.

[20]VICODIN *(hydrocodone + acetaminophen)*

▶LK ✪ ♀C ▶? ©II $$$
WARNING – Multiple strengths; see FORMS and write specific product on Rx.
ADULT – Moderate pain: 5/300 mg (max dose 8 tabs/day) and 7.5/300 mg (max dose of 6 tabs/day): 1–2 tabs PO q4–6h prn. 10/300 mg: 1 tab PO q4–6h prn (max of 6 tabs/day).
PEDS – Not approved in children.
FORMS – Generic/Trade: Tabs Vicodin (5/300), Vicodin ES (7.5/300), Vicodin HP (10/300) mg hydrocodone/mg acetaminophen, scored.

[20]LORTAB *(hydrocodone + acetaminophen)*

▶LK ✪ ♀C ▶? ©II $$
WARNING – Multiple strengths; see FORMS and write specific product on Rx.
ADULT – Moderate pain: 1–2 tabs 2.5/325 and 5/325 PO q4–6h prn, max dose 8 tabs/day. 1 tab 7.5/325 and 10/325 PO q4–6h prn, max dose 5 tabs/day.
PEDS – Not approved in children.

FORMS – Generic/Trade: Lortab 5/325 (scored), Lortab 7.5/325 (trade scored), Lortab 10/325 mg hydrocodone/mg acetaminophen. Generic only: Tabs 2.5/325 mg.

MOA – Serious: Respiratory depression/arrest, hepatotoxicity. Frequent: N/V, constipation, sedation.

[20]LORCET *(hydrocodone + acetaminophen)*

▶LK ⊗ ♀C ▶? ©II $$

WARNING – Multiple strengths; see FORMS and write specific product on Rx.

ADULT – Moderate pain: 1–2 caps (5/325) PO q4–6h prn, max dose 8 caps/day. 1 tab PO q4–6h prn (7.5/325 and 10/325), max dose 6 tabs/day.

PEDS – Not approved in children.

FORMS – Generic/Trade: Tabs, 5/325, 7.5/325,10/325 mg.

[21]VICOPROFEN *(hydrocodone + ibuprofen)*

▶LK ⊗ ♀– ▶? ©II $$

ADULT – Moderate pain: 1 tab PO q4–6h prn, max dose 5 tabs/day.

PEDS – Not approved in children.

FORMS – Generic only: Tabs 2.5/200, 5/200,7.5/200, 10/200 mg hydrocodone/ibuprofen.

NOTES – See NSAIDs: Other subclass warning.

MOA – Combination analgesic.

ADVERSE EFFECTS – Serious: Respiratory depression/arrest, hypersensitivity, GI bleeding, nephrotoxicity. Frequent: N/V, constipation, dyspepsia, sedation.

[22]PERCOCET *(oxycodone + acetaminophen, Percocet-Demi, Oxycocet, Endocet)*

▶L ⊗ ♀C ▶ – ©II $

WARNING – Multiple strengths; see FORMS and write specific product on Rx.

ADULT – Moderate to severe pain: 1–2 tabs PO q4–6h prn (2.5/325 and 5/325 mg). 1 tab PO q4–6h prn (7.5/325 and 10/325 mg).

PEDS – Not approved in children.

FORMS – Generic/Trade: Oxycodone/acetaminophen tabs 2.5/325, 5/325, 7.5/325, 10/325 mg. Trade only: (Primlev) tabs 2.5/300, 5/300, 7.5/300, 10/300 mg. Generic only: 10/325 mg.

[22]ROXICET *(oxycodone + acetaminophen)*

▶L ⊗ ♀C ▶ – ©II $

WARNING – Multiple strengths; see FORMS and write specific product on Rx.

ADULT – Moderate to severe pain: 1 tab PO q6h prn. Oral soln: 5 mL PO q6h prn.

PEDS – Not approved in children.

FORMS – Generic/Trade: Tabs 5/325 mg. Caps/caplets 5/325 mg. Soln 5/325 per 5 mL mg oxycodone/acetaminophen.

BURNS

Inpatient Analgesics (in the ED)	Outpatient Analgesics (discharge)
Non-Opioid	**Non-Opioid**
<u>Oral/Topical Analgesics (Mild to Moderate Pain):</u> [1]**Acetaminophen:** 500 mg, best if combined with NSAIDs [2]**Ibuprofen:** 400 mg, or [3]**Naproxen:** 500 mg, or [4]**Diclofenac:** 50 mg, or [5]**Ketorolac:** 10 mg [6]**Topical Diclofenac Gel:** thin layer to the affected area [7]**Topical Lidocaine** (2% cream): thin layer to the affected area <u>Regional Anesthesia and Analgesia (for musculoskeletal burns, chest wall and abdominal wall burns (Serratus Anterior Block (SAB) and Transversus Abdominis Block (TAP):</u> [8]**Bupivacaine w/o Epinephrine:** 0.25–0.5%, max 2.5 mg/kg	[2]**PO Ibuprofen:** 400 mg q8h × 3 days (max 5 days with 1200 mg/d) [3]**PO Naproxen:** 500 mg q12h × 3 days (max 5 days) [4]**PO Diclofenac:** 50 mg q8h × 3 days (max 5 days) [5]**PO Ketorolac:** 10 mg daily (analgesics ceiling dose) (max 5 days). [1]**PO Acetaminophen:** 500 mg PO q8h (max 1500 mg/day). Best if combined with [2]**Ibuprofen** at 400 mg q8h or [3]**Naproxen** at 500 mg q12h. [6]**Topical Diclofenac Gel:** Apply thin layer to affected area q12h for 5–7 days. [7]**Topical Lidocaine** (2% cream): up to two patches to the affected area

(continues)

Inpatient Analgesics (in the ED)	Outpatient Analgesics (discharge)
[8]**Bupivacaine w/ Epinephrine:** 0.25–0.5%, max 3.0 mg/kg [9]**Lidocaine w/o Epinephrine:** 0.5–2%, 4.5 mg/kg, max 300 mg [9]**Lidocaine w/ Epinephrine:** 0.5–2%, 7 mg/kg, max 500 mg [10]**Chloroprocaine:** 2–3%, max 11 mg/kg **Parenteral Regimen (Severe Pain):** [5]**IV Ketorolac:**10–15 mg IVP (analgesic ceiling dose) [9]**IV Lidocaine:** 1.5 mg/kg of 2% (preservative-free lidocaine - cardiac or pre-made bags only) over 15 min (max dose 200 mg [1]**IV Acetaminophen (APAP):** 1 g over 15 min (as adjunct to opioid/non-opioid) if patients are NPO/NPR or contraindications to opioids, NSAIDs, lidocaine, or ketamine [11]**Ketamine (Subdissociative Dose, SDK)** • **IV:** 0.3 mg/kg over 15 min, +/– continuous IV infusion at 0.15–0.2 mg/kg/h	

(continues)

Inpatient Analgesics (in the ED)	Outpatient Analgesics (discharge)
• **SQ:** 0.3 mg/kg over 15 min, +/− continuous SQ infusion at 0.15–0.2 mg/kg/h • **Intranasal (IN):** 0.5–1 mg/kg (weight-based) q5–10 min (consider using highly concentrated solutions: Adults:100 mg/mL Peds: 50 mg/mL. No more than 0.3–0.5 mL/per nostril) [12]**Dexmedetomidine:** IV: 0.5–1 µg/kg over 10–15 min (bolus); 0.1–0.2 µg/kg/h continuous infusion (range 0.1–1 µg/kg/h) with titration as needed	
Opioid	**Opioid**
<u>Oral Regimen:</u> [13]**Morphine:** Morphine Sulfate Immediate Release (MSIR): 15 mg [14]**Fentanyl:** Transbuccal 100–200 µg dissolvable tablets, repeat at 30–60 minutes if pain persists [15]**Hydromorphone:** 2 mg	**Opioids (in order of lesser degree of euphoria):** [13]**Morphine Sulfate Immediate Release (MSIR):** 15 mg q6–8h × 2–3 days (opioid-naïve patients)

(continues)

Inpatient Analgesics (in the ED)	Outpatient Analgesics (discharge)
Parenteral Regimen: [13]**Morphine:** **IV:** 0.05–0.1 mg/kg (weight-based), titrate q10–20 min • **IV:** 4–6 mg (fixed), titrate q10–20 min • **SQ:** 4–6 mg (fixed), re-administer as needed at q30–40 min • **IM:** 4–6 mg (fixed), re-administer as needed at q30–40 min (IM route should be avoided due to pain upon injection, muscle fibrosis, necrosis, increase in dosing requirements) **Nebulized** (via Breath Actuated Nebulizer [BAN]: Adults: 10–20 mg (fixed), repeat q15–20 min up to three doses Peds: 0.2–0.4 mg/kg (weight-based), repeat q15–20 min up to three doses • **PCA:** Demand dose: 1–2 mg Continuous basal infusion: 0.5–2 mg/h	[17]**Hydrocodone/Acetaminophen (Norco)** 5/325 mg: 1–2 tabs q6–8h × 2–3 days [18]**Hydrocodone/Acetaminophen (Vicodin, Lortab, Lorcet)** 5/300 mg: 1–2 tabs q6–8h × 2–3 days [19]**Hydrocodone/Ibuprofen (Vicoprofen)** 5/200 mg: 1–2 tabs q6–8h × 2–3 days [20]**Oxycodone/Acetaminophen (Percocet, Roxicet)** 5/325 mg: 1–2 tabs q6–8h × 2–3 days [15]**Hydromorphone:** 2–4 mg q6–8h × 2–3 days (for opioid-naïve patients start with 2 mg dose)

(continues)

Inpatient Analgesics (in the ED)	Outpatient Analgesics (discharge)

[14]Fentanyl:
• **IV:** 0.25–0.1 µg/kg (weight-based), titrate q10 min
• **IV:** 50–100 µg (fixed), titrate q10–20 min
  Nebulized (via BAN):
  Adults: 2–4 µg/kg (weight-based), titrate q20–30 min, up to three doses
  Peds: 2–4 µg/kg (weight-based), titrate q20–30 min, up to three doses
• **Intranasal (IN):** 1–2 µg/kg (weight-based), titrate q5–10 min (consider using highly concentrated solutions:
  Adults: 100 µg/mL
  Peds: 50 µg/mL. No more than 0.3–0.5 mL/per nostril)
• **Transmucosal:** 15–20 mcg/kg lollipops
• **PCA:**
  Demand dose: 20–50 µg
  Continuous basal infusion: 0.05–0.1 µg/kg/h	

BURNS

(continues)

Inpatient Analgesics (in the ED)	Outpatient Analgesics (discharge)

[15]**Hydromorphone:**
• **IV:** 0.5–1 mg initial, titrate q10–15 min
• **SQ:** 0.5–2 mg, titrate q30–40 min
• **IM:** 0.5–2 mg, titrate q30–40 min (IM route should be avoided due to pain, muscle fibrosis, necrosis, increase in dosing requirements)
• **PCA:**
  Demand dose: 0.2–0.4 mg
  Continuous basal infusion: 0.1–0.4 mg/h
[16]**Sufentanil:**
• **Intranasal (IN):** 0.5 µg/kg, titration q10 min up to three doses	

[1]**ACETAMINOPHEN** *(Tylenol, Panadol, Tempra, Ofirmev, Paracetamol, Abenol, Atasol, Pediatrix)*

▶ LK ♀B ▶+ $

ADULT — Analgesic/antipyretic: 325–1000 mg PO q4–6h pm. 650 mg PR q4–6h pm. Max dose 4 g/day. OA: Extended-release: 2 caps PO q8h around the clock. Max dose 6 caps/day.

PEDS — Analgesic/antipyretic: 10–15 mg/kg q4–6h PO/PR pm. Max 5 doses/day.

UNAPPROVED ADULT — OA: 1000 mg PO four times per day.

FORMS — OTC: Tabs 325, 500, 650 mg. Chewable tabs 80 mg. Orally disintegrating tabs 80, 160 mg. Caps/gelcaps 500 mg. Extended-release caplets 650 mg. Liquid 160 mg/5 mL, 500 mg/15 mL. Supps 80, 120, 325, 650 mg.

[2]IBUPROFEN (Motrin, Advil, Nuprin, Rufen, NeoProfen, Caldolor)

▶L ⊗ ♀B (D in 3rd trimester) ▶+ ■

ADULT — RA/OA, gout: 200–800 mg PO three to four times per day. Mild to moderate pain: 400 mg PO q4–6h. 400–800 mg IV (Caldolor) q6h prn. 400 mg IV (Caldolor) q4–6h or 100–200 mg q4h prn. Primary dysmenorrhea: 400 mg PO q4h prn. Fever: 200 mg PO q4–6h prn. Migraine pain: 200–400 mg PO, not to exceed 400 mg in 24 h unless directed by a physician (OTC dosing). Max dose 3.2 g/day.

PEDS — JRA: 30–50 mg/kg/day PO divided q6h. Max dose 2400 mg/24 h. 20 mg/kg/day may be adequate for milder disease. Analgesic/antipyretic, age older than 6 mo: 5–10 mg/kg PO q6–8h prn. Max dose 40 mg/kg/day. Patent ductus arteriosus in neonates 32 weeks' gestational age or younger weighing 500–1500 g (NeoProfen): Specialized dosing.

FORMS — OTC: Caps/Liqui-Gel caps 200 mg. Tabs 100, 200 mg. Chewable tabs 100 mg. Susp (infant gtts) 50 mg/1.25 mL (with calibrated dropper), 100 mg/5 mL. Rx Generic/Trade: Tabs 400, 600, 800 mg.

NOTES — May antagonize antiplatelet effects of aspirin if given simultaneously. Take aspirin 2 h prior to ibuprofen. Administer IV (Caldolor) over at least 30 min; hydration important.

MOA — Anti-inflammatory/antipyretic, analgesic.

ADVERSE EFFECTS — Serious: Hypersensitivity, GI bleeding, nephrotoxicity. Frequent: Nausea, dyspepsia.

[3]NAPROXEN (Naprosyn, Aleve, Anaprox, EC-Naprosyn, Naprelan, Prevacid, NapraPAC)

▶L ✪ ♀B (D in 3rd trimester) ▶+ $■

WARNING — Multiple strengths; see FORMS and write specific product on Rx.

ADULT — RA/OA, ankylosing spondylitis, pain, dysmenorrhea, acute tendinitis and bursitis, fever: 250–500 mg PO two times per day. Delayed-release: 375–500 mg PO two times per day (do not crush or chew). Controlled-release: 750–1000 mg PO daily. Acute gout: 750 mg PO once, then 250 mg PO q8h until the attack subsides. Controlled-release: 1000–1500 mg PO once, then 1000 mg PO daily until the attack subsides.

PEDS — JRA: 10–20 mg/kg/day PO divided two times per day (up to 1250 mg/24 h). Pain for age older than 2 yo: 5–7 mg/kg/dose PO q8–12 h.

UNAPPROVED ADULT — Acute migraine: 750 mg PO once, then 250–500 mg PO pm. Migraine prophylaxis, menstrual migraine: 500 mg PO two times per day beginning 1 day prior to onset of menses and ending on last day of period.

FORMS — OTC Generic/Trade (Aleve): Tabs, immediate-release 200 mg. OTC Trade only (Aleve): Caps, Gelcaps, immediate-release 200 mg. Rx Generic/Trade: Tabs, immediate-release (Naprosyn) 250, 375, 500 mg. (Anaprox) 275, 550 mg. Tabs, delayed-release enteric-coated (EC-Naprosyn) 375, 500 mg. Tabs, controlled-release (Naprelan) 375, 500, 750 mg. Susp (Naprosyn) 125 mg/5 mL. Prevacid NapraPAC: 7 lansoprazole 15 mg caps packaged with 14 naproxen tabs 375 mg or 500 mg.

NOTES — All dosing is based on naproxen content: 500 mg naproxen is equivalent to 550 mg naproxen sodium.

MOA — Anti-inflammatory, analgesic.

ADVERSE EFFECTS — Serious: Hypersensitivity, GI bleeding, nephrotoxicity. Frequent: Nausea, dyspepsia.

[4]DICLOFENAC (Voltaren, Voltaren XR, Flector, Zipsor, Cambia, Zorvolex, Voltaren Rapide)

▶L ⊗ ♀B (D in 3rd trimester) ▶ – $$$■

WARNING — Multiple strengths; see FORMS and write specific product on Rx.

ADULT — OA: Immediate- or delayed-release: 50 mg PO two to three times per day or 75 mg two times per day. Extended-release 100 mg PO daily. Gel: Apply 4 g to knees or 2 g to hands four times per day using enclosed dosing card. RA: Immediate- or delayed-release 50 mg PO three to four times per day or 75 mg two times per day. Extended-release 100 mg PO one to two times per day. Ankylosing spondylitis: Immediate- or delayed-release 25 mg PO four times per day and at bedtime. Analgesia and primary dysmenorrhea: Immediate- or delayed-release 50 mg PO three times per day. Acute pain in strains, sprains, or contusions: Apply 1 patch to painful area two times per day. Acute migraine with or without aura: 50 mg single dose (Cambia), mix packet with 30–60 mL water.

PEDS — Not approved in children.

UNAPPROVED PEDS — JRA: 2–3 mg/kg/day PO.

FORMS – Generic/Trade: Tabs, extended-release (Voltaren XR) 100 mg. Topical gel (Voltaren) 1% 100 g tube. Generic only: Tabs, immediate-release: 25, 50 mg. Generic only: Tabs, delayed-release: 25, 50, 75 mg. Trade only: Patch (Flector) 1.3% diclofenac epolamine. Trade only: Caps, liquid-filled (Zipsor) 25 mg. Caps (Zorvolex) 18, 35 mg. Trade only: Powder for oral soln (Cambia) 50 mg.

NOTES – Check LFTs at baseline, within 4–8 weeks of initiation, then periodically. Do not apply patch to damaged or nonintact skin. Wash hands, and avoid eye contact when handling the patch. Do not wear patch while bathing or showering.

MOA – Anti-inflammatory, analgesic.

ADVERSE EFFECTS – Serious: Hypersensitivity, GI bleeding, hepato/nephrotoxicity. Frequent: Nausea, dyspepsia, pruritus and dermatitis with patch and gel.

[5]KETOROLAC *(Toradol)*

▶L ⊗ ♀B (D in 3rd trimester) ▶+ $$■

WARNING – Indicated for short-term (up to 5 days) therapy only. Ketorolac is a potent NSAID and can cause serious GI and renal adverse effects. It may also increase the risk of bleeding by inhibiting platelet function. Contraindicated in patients with active peptic ulcer disease, recent GI bleeding or perforation, a history of peptic ulcer disease or GI bleeding, or advanced renal impairment.

ADULT – Moderately severe, acute pain, single-dose treatment: 30–60 mg IM or 15–30 mg IV. Multiple-dose treatment: 15–30 mg IV/IM q6 h. IV/IM doses are not to exceed 60 mg/day for age 65 yo or older, wt < 50 kg, and patients with moderately elevated serum creatinine. Oral continuation therapy: 1.0 mg PO q4–6h prn, max dose 40 mg/day. Combined duration IV/IM and PO is not to exceed 5 days.

PEDS – Not approved in children.

UNAPPROVED PEDS – Pain: 0.5 mg/kg/dose IM/IV q6h (up to 30 mg q6h or 120 mg/day), give 10 mg PO qGh pm (up to 40 mg/day) for wt > 50 kg.

FORMS – Generic only: Tabs 10 mg.

MOA – Serious: Hypersensitivity, GI bleeding, nephrotoxicity. Frequent: Nausea, dyspepsia.

[6]DICLOFENAC—TOPICAL *(Solaraze, Voltaren, Pennsaid)*

▶L ♀C Category D at 30 weeks gestation and beyond. Avoid use starting at 30 weeks gestation. ▶? $$$■

WARNING – Risk of cardiovascular and GI events.

ADULT – Osteoarthritis of areas amenable to topical therapy: 2 g (upper extremities) to 4 g (lower extremities) four times per day (Voltaren); 40 gtts to knee(s) four times daily.

PEDS – Not approved in children.

FORMS – Generic/Trade: Gel 3% (Solaraze) 100 g. Soln 1.5% (Pennsaid) 150 mL. Trade only: Gel 1% (Voltaren) 100 g. Soln 2.0% Pump (Pennsaid) 112 g.

NOTES – Avoid exposure to sun and sunlamps. Use caution in aspirin-sensitive patients. When using for OA (Voltaren), max daily dose 16 g to any single lower extremity joint, 8 g to any single upper-extremity joint. Avoid use in setting of aspirin allergy or CABG surgery.

MOA – Inhibits prostaglandins at level of cyclooxygenase.

ADVERSE EFFECTS – Frequent: Rash, abdominal cramps, nausea, indigestion.

BURNS

[7]LIDOCAINE—TOPICAL (Xylocaine, Lidoderm, Numby Stuff, LMX, Zingo, Maxilene)

▶LK ♀B ▶+ $

WARNING – Contraindicated in allergy to amide-type anesthetics.

ADULT – Topical anesthesia: Apply to affected area prn. Dose varies with anesthetic procedure, degree of anesthesia required, and individual patient response. Post-herpetic neuralgia (patch): Apply up to 3 patches to affected area at once for up to 12 h within a 24 h period.

PEDS – Topical anesthesia: Apply to affected area prn. Dose varies with anesthetic procedure, degree of anesthesia required, and individual patient response. Max 3 mg/kg/dose, do not repeat dose within 2 h. Intradermal powder injection for venipuncture/IV cannulation, for age 3–18 yo (Zingo): 0.5 mg to site 1–10 min prior.

UNAPPROVED PEDS – Topical anesthesia prior to venipuncture: Apply 30 min prior to procedure (ELA-Max 4%).

FORMS – For membranes of mouth and pharynx: Spray 10%, oint 5%, liquid 5%, soln 2%, 4% dental patch. For urethral use: Jelly 2%. Patch (Lidoderm $$$$$) 5%. Intradermal powder injection system: 0.5 mg (Zingo). OTC Trade only: Liposomal lidocaine 4% (ELA-Max).

NOTES – Apply patches only to intact skin to cover the most painful area. Patches may be cut into smaller sizes with scissors prior to removal of the release liner. Store and dispose out of the reach of children and pets to avoid possible toxicity from ingestion.

MOA – Anesthetic.

ADVERSE EFFECTS – Frequent: Skin irritation. Severe: CNS effects, bradycardia, bronchospasm, hypotension, allergic reactions.

[8]BUPIVACAINE *(Marcaine, Sensorcaine)*

▶LK ♀C ▶? $■

ADULT – Local anesthesia, nerve block: 0.25% injection. Up to 2.5 mg/kg without epinephrine and up 3.0 mg/kg with epinephrine.

PEDS – Not recommended in children younger than 12 yo.

FORMS – 0.25%, 0.5%, 0.75%, all with or without epinephrine.

NOTES – Onset 5 min, duration 2–4 h (longer with epi). Amide group.

MOA – Amide local anesthetic.

ADVERSE EFFECTS – Serious: Seizures, cardiovascular depression, bradycardia, hypersensitivity, methemoglobinemia. Frequent: None.

[9]LIDOCAINE—LOCAL ANESTHETIC *(Xylocaine)*

▶LK ♀B ▶? $

ADULT – Without epinephrine: Max dose 4.5 mg/kg not to exceed 300 mg. With epinephrine: Max dose 7 mg/kg not to exceed 500 mg. Dose for regional block varies by region.

PEDS – Same as adult.

FORMS – 0.5, 1, 1.5, 2%. With epi: 0.5, 1, 1.5, 2%.

NOTES – Onset within 2 min, duration 30–60 min (longer with epi). Amide group. Use "cardiac lidocaine" (ie, IV formulation) for Bier blocks at max dose of 3 mg/kg so that neither epinephrine nor methylparaben are injected IV.

MOA – Amide local anesthetic.

ADVERSE EFFECTS – Serious: Seizures, cardiovascular depression, bradycardia, hypersensitivity, methemoglobinemia. Frequent: None.

[10]CHLOROPROCAINE *(Nesacaine)*

▶LK ♀C ▶? $

ADULT – Epidural anesthesia: 18–24 mL of 2.0–3.0% chloroprocaine will provide 30–60 min of surgical anesthesia. Infiltration and peripheral nerve block: 0.5–40 mL of 1–3% chloroprocaine.

PEDS – Same as adult, age 3 yo or older.

FORMS – 1, 2, 3%.

NOTES – Max local dose: 11 mg/kg.

MOA – Ester local anesthetic.

ADVERSE EFFECTS – Serious: Seizures, cardiovascular depression, bradycardia, hypersensitivity, methemoglobinemia. Frequent: None.

[11]KETAMINE *(Ketalar)*

▶L ♀C ▶? ©III $■

WARNING – Post-anesthetic emergence reactions up to 24 h later manifested as dreamlike state, vivid imagery, hallucinations, and delirium reported in about 12% of cases. Incidence reduced when (1) age less than 15 yo or greater than 65 yo, (2) concomitant use of benzodiazepines, lower dose, or used as induction agent only (because of use of post-intubation sedation).

ADULT – Induction of anesthesia: Adult: 1–2 mg/kg IV over 1–2 min (produces 5–10 min dissociative state) or 6.5–13 mg/kg IM (produces 10–20 min dissociative state).

PEDS – Age over 16 yo: same as adult.

UNAPPROVED ADULT – Dissociative sedation: 1–2 mg/kg IV over 1–2 mm (sedation lasting 10–20 min); repeat 0.5 mg/kg doses every 5–15 min may be given; 4–5 mg/kg IM (sedation lasting 15–30 min); repeat 2–4 mg/kg IM can be given if needed after 10–15 min. Analgesia adjunct subdissociative dose: 0.01–0.5 mg/kg in conjunction with opioid analgesia.

UNAPPROVED PEDS – Dissociative sedation: Age older than 3 mo: 1–2 mg/kg IV (produces 5–10 min dissociative state) over 1–2 min or 4–5 mg/kg IM (produces 10–20 min dissociative state). Not approved for age younger than 3 mo.

FORMS – Generic/Trade: 10, 50, 100 mg/mL.

NOTES – Recent evidence suggests ketamine is not contraindicated in patients with head injuries. However, avoid if CAD or severe HTN. Concurrent administration of atropine no longer recommended. Consider prophylactic ondansetron to reduce vomiting and prophylactic midazolam (0.3 mg/kg) to reduce recovery reactions.

MOA – NMDA receptor antagonist that produces dissociative state.

ADVERSE EFFECTS – Serious: Laryngospasm, hallucinatory emergence reactions, hypersalivation. Frequent: Nystagmus, hypertension, tachycardia; N/V, muscular hypertonicity, myoclonus.

[12]DEXMEDETOMIDINE (Precedex)

▶LK ♀C ▶? $$$

ADULT – ICU sedation less than 24 h: Load 1 mcg/kg over 10 min followed by infusion 0.6 mcg/kg/h (ranges from 0.2–1.0 mcg/kg/h) titrated to desired sedation endpoint. Procedural sedation: Load 1 mcg/kg over 10 min followed by infusion of 0.6 mcg/kg/h titrated up or down to clinical effect in range of 0.2–1 mcg/kg/h depending on procedure and patient (0.7 mcg/kg/h for fiberoptic intubation). Reduce dose in impaired hepatic function and geriatric patients.

PEDS – Not recommended age younger than 18 yo.

NOTES — Alpha-2 adrenergic agonist with sedative properties. Beware of bradycardia and hypotension. Avoid in advanced heart block.

MOA — Alpha-2 adrenergic agonist with sedative properties.

[13]MORPHINE *(MS Contin, Kadian, Avinza, Roxanol, Oramorph SR, MSIR, DepoDur, Statex, M.O.S. Doloral, M-Eslon)*

▶L ♀C ▶? ©III $■

WARNING — Multiple strengths; see FORMS and write specific product on Rx. Drinking alcohol while taking Avinza may result in a rapid release of a potentially fatal dose of morphine.

ADULT — Moderate to severe pain: 10–30 mg PO q4h (immediate-release tabs, or oral soln). Controlled-release (MS Contin, Oramorph SR): 30 mg PO q8–12 h. (Kadian): 20 mg PO q12–24h. Extended-release caps (Avinza): 30 mg PO daily: 10 mg q4h IM/SC: 2.5–15 mg/70 kg IV over 4–5 min: 10–20 mg PR q4h. Pain with major surgery (DepoDur): 10–15 mg once epidurally at the lumbar level prior to surgery (max dose 20 mg), or 10 mg epidurally after clamping of the umbilical cord with cesarean section.

PEDS — Moderate to severe pain: 0.1–0.2 mg/kg up to 15 mg IM/SC/IV q2–4h.

UNAPPROVED PEDS — Moderate to severe pain: 0.2–0.5 mg/kg/dose PO (immediate-release) q4–6h; 0.3–0.6 mg/kg/dose PO (controlled-release) q12h.

FORMS — Generic only: Tabs, immediate-release 15, 30 mg ($). Oral soln 10 mg/5 mL, 20 mg/5 mL, 20 mg/mL (concentrate). Rectal supps 5, 10, 20, 30 mg. Generic/Trade: Controlled-release tabs (MS Contin) 15, 30, 60, 100, 200 mg

($$$$). Controlled-release caps (Kadian) 10, 20, 30, 50, 60, 80, 100 mg ($$$$$). Extended-release caps (Avinza) 30, 45, 60, 75, 90, 120 mg. Trade only: Controlled-release caps (Kadian) 40, 200 mg.

NOTES – Titrate dose as high as necessary to relieve cancer or nonmalignant pain where chronic opioids are necessary. The active metabolites may accumulate in hepatic/renal insufficiency and the elderly leading to increased analgesic and sedative effects. Do not break, chew, or crush MS Contin or Oramorph SR. Kadian and Avinza caps may be opened and sprinkled in applesauce for easier administration; however, the pellets should not be crushed or chewed. Doses more than 1600 mg/day of Avinza contain a potentially nephrotoxic quantity of fumaric acid. Do not mix DepoDur with other medications; do not administer any other medications into epidural space for at least 48 h. Severe opiate overdose with respiratory depression has occurred with intrathecal leakage of DepoDur.

MOA – Opioid agonist analgesic.

ADVERSE EFFECTS – Serious: Respiratory depression/arrest. Frequent: N/V, constipation, sedation, hypotension.

[14]FENTANYL *(IONSYS, Duragesic, Actiq, Fentora, Sublimaze, Abstral, Subsys, Lazanda, Onsolis)*

▶L ♀C ▶? ©III $■

WARNING – Duragesic patches, Actiq, Fentora, Abstral, Subsys, and Lazanda are contraindicated in the management of acute or postop pain due to potentially life-threatening respiratory depression in opioid nontolerant patients. Instruct patients and their caregivers that even used patches/lozenges on a stick can be fatal to a child or pet. Dispose via toilet. Actiq and Fentora are not interchangeable. IONSYS: For hospital use only; remove prior to discharge. Can cause life-threatening respiratory depression.

ADULT – Duragesic patches: Chronic pain: 12–100 mcg/h patch q72 h. Titrate dose to the needs of the patient. Some patients require q48h dosing. May wear more than 1 patch to achieve the correct analgesic effect. Actiq: Breakthrough cancer pain: 200–1600 mcg sucked over 15 min; if 200 mcg ineffective for 6 units use higher strength. Goal is 4 lozenges on a stick/day in conjunction with long-acting opioid. Buccal tab (Fentora) for breakthrough cancer pain: 100–800 mcg, titrated to pain relief; may repeat once after 30 min during single episode of breakthrough pain. See prescribing information for dose conversion from transmucosal lozenges. Buccal soluble film (Onsolis) for breakthrough cancer pain: 200–1200 mcg titrated to pain relief; no more than 4 doses/day separated by at least 2 h. Postop analgesia: 50–100 mcg IM; repeat in 1–2 h prn. SL tab (Abstral) for breakthrough cancer pain: 100 mcg, may repeat once after 30 min. Specialized titration. SL spray (Subsys) for breakthrough cancer pain 100 mcg, may repeat once after 30 min. Specialized titration. Nasal spray (Lazanda) for breakthrough cancer pain: 100 mcg. Specialized titration. IONSYS: Acute postop pain: Specialized dosing.

PEDS – Transdermal (Duragesic): Not approved in children younger than 2 yo or in opioid-naïve. Use adult dosing for age older than 2 yo. Children converting to a 25-mcg patch should be receiving 45 mg or more oral morphine equivalents/day. Actiq: Not approved for age younger than 16 yo. IONSYS not approved in children. Abstral, Subsys, and Lazanda: Not approved for age younger than 18 yo.

UNAPPROVED ADULT – Analgesia/procedural sedation/labor analgesia: 50–100 mcg IV or IM q1–2h prn.

UNAPPROVED PEDS – Analgesia: 1–2 mcg/kg/dose IV/IM q30–60 min prn or continuous IV infusion 1–3 mcg/kg/h (not to exceed adult dosing). Procedural sedation: 2–3 mcg/kg/dose for age 1–3 yo; 1–2 mcg/kg/dose for age 3–12 yo, 0.5–1 mcg/kg/dose (not to exceed adult dosing) for age older than 12 yo, procedural sedation doses may be repeated q30–60 min prn.

FORMS – Generic/Trade: Transdermal patches 12, 25, 50, 75, 100 mcg/h. Actiq lozenges on a stick, berry-flavored 200, 400, 600, 800, 1200, 1600 mcg. Trade only: (Fentora) buccal tab 100, 200, 400, 600, 800 mcg, packs of 4 or 28 tabs. Trade only: (Onsolis) buccal soluble film 200, 400, 600, 800, 1200 mcg in child-resistant, protective foil, packs of 30 films. Trade only: (Abstral) SL tabs 100, 200, 300, 400, 600, 800 mcg, packs of 4 or 32 tabs. Trade only: (Subsys) SL spray 100, 200, 400, 600, 800, 1200, 1600 mcg blister packs in cartons of 10 and 30 (30 only for 1200 and 1600 mcg). Trade only: (Lazanda) nasal spray 100, 400 mcg/spray, 8 sprays/bottle.

NOTES – Do not use patches for acute pain or in opioid-naïve patients. Oral transmucosal fentanyl doses of 5 mcg/kg provide effects similar to 0.75–1.25 mcg/kg of fentanyl IM. Lozenges on a stick should be sucked, not chewed. Flush lozenge remnants (without stick) down the toilet. For transdermal systems: Apply patch to non-hairy skin. Clip (do not shave) hair if you have to apply to hairy area. Fever or external heat sources may increase fentanyl released from patch. Patch should be removed prior to MRI and reapplied after the test. Dispose of a used patch by folding with the adhesive side of the patch adhering to itself then flush it down the toilet immediately. Do not cut

the patch in half. For Duragesic patches and Actiq lozenges on a stick: Titrate dose as high as necessary to relieve cancer or nonmalignant pain where chronic opioids are necessary. Do not suck, chew, or swallow buccal tab. IONSYS: Apply to intact skin on the chest or upper arm. Each dose activated by the patient is delivered over a 10-min period. Remove prior to hospital discharge. Do not allow gel to touch mucous membranes. Dispose using gloves. Keep all forms of fentanyl out of the reach of children or pets. Concomitant use with potent CYP3A4 inhibitors such as ritonavir, ketoconazole, itraconazole, clarithromycin, nelfinavir, and nefazodone may result in an increase in fentanyl plasma concentrations, which could increase or prolong adverse drug effects and may cause potentially fatal respiratory depression. Onsolis is available only through the FOCUS Program and requires prescriber, pharmacy, and patient enrollment. Used films should be discarded into toilet. Abstral, Subsys, and Lazanda: Outpatients, prescribers, pharmacies, and distributors must be enrolled in TIRF REMS Access program before patient may receive medication.
MOA – Opioid agonist analgesic.
ADVERSE EFFECTS – Serious: Respiratory depression/arrest, chest wall rigidity. Frequent: N/V, constipation, sedation, skin irritation, dental decay with Actiq.

[15]HYDROMORPHONE *(Dilaudid, Exalgo, Hydromorph Contin)*

▶L ♀C ▷? ©III $■

ADULT – Moderate to severe pain: 2–4 mg PO q4–6h. Initial dose (opioid-naïve): 0.5–2 mg SC/IM or slow IV q4–6h prn. 3 mg PR q6–8h. Controlled-release tabs: 8–64 mg daily.

PEDS – Not approved in children.

UNAPPROVED PEDS – Pain age 12 yo or younger: 0.03–0.08 mg/kg PO q4–6h prn. 0.015 mg/kg/dose IV q4–6h prn, use adult dose for older than 12 yo.

FORMS – Generic/Trade: Tabs 2, 4, 8 mg (8 mg trade scored). Oral soln 5 mg/5 mL. Controlled-release tabs (Exalgo): 8, 12, 16, 32 mg.

NOTES – In opioid-naïve patients, consider an initial dose of 0.5 mg or less IM/SC/IV. SC/IM/IV doses after initial dose should be individualized. May be given by slow IV injection over 2–5 min. Titrate dose as high as necessary to relieve cancer or nonmalignant pain where chronic opioids are necessary. 1.5 mg IV = 75 mg PO. Exalgo intended for opioid-tolerant patients only.

MOA – Opioid agonist analgesic.

ADVERSE EFFECTS – Serious: Respiratory depression/arrest. Frequent: N/V, constipation, sedation.

[16]SUFENTANIL *(Sufenta)*

▶L ♀C ▶? ©III $ ■

ADULT – General anesthesia: Induction: 8–30 mcg/kg IV; maintenance 0.5–10 mcg/kg IV. Conscious sedation: Loading dose: 0.1–0.5 mcg/kg; maintenance infusion 0.005–0.01 mcg/kg/min

PEDS – General anesthesia: Induction: 8–30 mcg/kg IV; maintenance 0.5–10 mcg/kg 1V. Conscious sedation: Loading dose: 0.1–0.5 mcg/kg; maintenance infusion 0.005–0.01 mcg/kg/min.

MOA – Serious: Respiratory depression, hypotension, bradycardia, chest wall rigidity, opiate dependence, hypersensitivity. Frequent: Sedation, N/V.

[17]NORCO *(hydrocodone + acetaminophen)*

▶LK ✪ ♀C ▶? ©II $$

WARNING – Multiple strengths; see FORMS and write specific product on Rx.

ADULT – Moderate to severe pain: 1–2 tabs PO q4–6h prn (5/325), max dose 12 tabs/day. 1 tab (7.5/325 and 10/325) PO q4–6h prn, max dose 8 and 6 tabs/day, respectively.

PEDS – Not approved in children.

FORMS – Generic/Trade: Tabs 5/325, 7.5/325, 10/325 mg hydrocodone/acetaminophen, scored. Generic only: Soln 7.5/325 mg per 15 mL.

[18]VICODIN *(hydrocodone + acetaminophen)*

▶LK ✪ ♀C ▶? ©II $$$

WARNING – Multiple strengths; see FORMS and write specific product on Rx.

ADULT – Moderate pain: 5/300 mg (max dose 8 tabs/day) and 7.5/300 mg (max dose of 6 tabs/day): 1–2 tabs PO q4–6h prn. 10/300 mg: 1 tab PO q4–6h prn (max of 6 tabs/day).

PEDS – Not approved in children.

FORMS – Generic/Trade: Tabs Vicodin (5/300), Vicodin ES (7.5/300), Vicodin HP (10/300) mg hydrocodone/mg acetaminophen, scored.

[18]LORTAB *(hydrocodone + acetaminophen)*

▶LK ✪ ♀C ▶– ©II $$

WARNING – Multiple strengths; see FORMS and write specific product on Rx.

ADULT — Moderate pain: 1–2 tabs 2.5/325 and 5/325 PO q4–6h prn, max dose 8 tabs/day. 1 tab 7.5/325 and 10/325 PO q4–6h prn, max dose 5 tabs/day.

PEDS — Not approved in children.

FORMS — Generic/Trade: Lortab 5/325 (scored), Lortab 7.5/325 {trade scored}, Lortab 10/325 mg hydrocodone/mg acetaminophen. Generic only: Tabs 2.5/325 mg.

MOA — Serious: Respiratory depression/arrest, hepatotoxicity. Frequent: N/V, constipation, sedation.

[18]LORCET (hydrocodone + acetaminophen)

▶LK ⊗ ♀– ▶? ©II $$

WARNING — Multiple strengths; see FORMS and write specific product on Rx.

ADULT — Moderate pain: 1–2 caps (5/325) PO q4–6h prn, max dose 8 caps/day. 1 tab PO q4–6h prn (7.5/325 and 10/325), max dose 6 tabs/day.

PEDS — Not approved in children.

FORMS — Generic/Trade: Tabs, 5/325, 7.5/325,10/325 mg.

[19]VICOPROFEN (hydrocodone + ibuprofen)

▶LK ⊗ ♀– ▶? ©II $$

ADULT — Moderate pain: 1 tab PO q4–6h prn, max dose 5 tabs/day.

PEDS — Not approved in children.

FORMS — Generic only: Tabs 2.5/200, 5/200, 7.5/200, 10/200 mg hydrocodone/ibuprofen.

NOTES — See NSAIDs: Other subclass warning.

MOA — Combination analgesic.

ADVERSE EFFECTS – Serious: Respiratory depression/arrest, hypersensitivity, GI bleeding, nephrotoxicity. Frequent: N/V, constipation, dyspepsia, sedation.

[20]PERCOCET (oxycodone + acetaminophen, Percocet-Demi, Oxycocet, Endocet)

▶L ✪ ♀C ▶– ©II $

WARNING – Multiple strengths; see FORMS and write specific product on Rx.

ADULT – Moderate to severe pain: 1–2 tabs PO q4–6h prn (2.5/325 and 5/325 mg). 1 tab PO q4–6h prn (7.5/325 and 10/325 mg).

PEDS – Not approved in children.

FORMS – Generic/Trade: Oxycodone/acetaminophen tabs 2.5/325, 5/325, 7.5/325, 10/325 mg. Trade only: (Prim lev) tabs 2.5/300, 5/300, 7.5/300, 10/300 mg. Generic only: 10/325 mg.

[20]ROXICET (oxycodone + acetaminophen)

▶L ✪ ♀C ▶– ©II $

WARNING – Multiple strengths; see FORMS and write specific product on Rx.

ADULT – Moderate to severe pain: 1 tab PO q6h prn. Oral soln: 5 mL PO q6h prn.

PEDS – Not approved in children.

FORMS – Generic/Trade: Tabs 5/325 mg. Caps/caplets 5/325 mg. Soln 5/325 per 5 mL mg oxycodone/acetaminophen.

DENTAL PAIN

Inpatient Analgesics (in the ED)	Outpatient Analgesics (discharge)
Non-Opioid	**Non-Opioid**
Oral/Topical Analgesics: [1]**Ibuprofen:** 400 mg, or [2]**Naproxen:** 500 mg, or [3]**Diclofenac:** 50 mg, or [4]**Ketorolac:** 10 mg [5]**Acetaminophen:** 500–1000 mg, best if combined with NSAIDs [6]**Oraquix** (prilocaine + lidocaine) gel, applied topically **Dental Block:** [7]**Articane:** 4%, max 7 mg/kg [8]**Bupivacaine** w/o epi: 0.25–0.5%, max 2.5 mg/kg [8]**Bupivacaine** with epi: 0.25–0.5%, max 3.0 mg/kg [9]**Lidocaine** w/o epi: 0.5–2%, 4.5 mg/kg, max 300 mg [9]**Lidocaine** with epi: 0.5–2%, 7 mg/kg, max 500 mg [10]**Mepivacaine:** 1–2%, max 5 mg/kg	[1]**PO Ibuprofen:** 400 mg q8h × 3 days (max 5 days with 1200 mg/d) [2]**PO Naproxen:** 500 mg q12h × 3 days (max 5 days) [3]**PO Diclofenac:** 50 mg q8h × 3 days (max 5 days) [5]**PO Acetaminophen:** 500 mg PO q8h × 3 days (max 1500 mg/day). Best if combined with [1]**Ibuprofen** at 400 mg q8h

(*continues*)

Inpatient Analgesics (in the ED)	Outpatient Analgesics (discharge)
Non-Opioid	**Non-Opioid**
[11]**Prilocaine:** 4%, max 5 mg/kg w/o epi, 7 mg/kg with epi. [12]**Procaine:** 0.25–0.5%, max 6 mg/kg [13]**Ropivacaine:** 0.2–1%, max 3 mg/kg	
Opioid	**Opioid**
Opioids should not be routinely used in the ED for dental pain. Their use should be limited to patients with severe traumatic dental pain, intractable pain, and in cases of failed non-opioid analgesia, including dental block. When these agents are used, lowest effective dose must be used. [14]**Morphine Sulfate Immediate Release (MSIR):** 15 mg PO	Opioids should not be routinely used at discharge for dental pain. Their use should be limited to patients with severe traumatic dental pain, intractable pain, and in cases of failed non-opioid analgesia. When these agents are used, lowest effective dose and shortest treatment course must be used. [14]**Morphine Sulfate Immediate Release (MSIR):** 15 mg q6–8h × 2–3 days (opioid-naïve patients)

(continues)

Inpatient Analgesics (in the ED)	Outpatient Analgesics (discharge)
Opioid	Opioid
[15]Hydrocodone/Acetaminophen (Norco) 5/325 mg: 1–2 tabs PO	[15]Hydrocodone/Acetaminophen (Norco) 5/325 mg: 1–2 tabs q6–8h × 2–3 days
[16]Hydrocodone/Acetaminophen (Vicodin, Lortab, Lorcet) 5/300 mg: 1–2 tabs PO	[16]Hydrocodone/Acetaminophen (Vicodin, Lortab, Lorcet) 5/300 mg: 1–2 tabs q6–8h × 2–3 days
[17]Hydrocodone/Ibuprofen (Vicoprofen) 5/200 mg: 1–2 tabs PO	[17]Hydrocodone/Ibuprofen (Vicoprofen) 5/200 mg: 1–2 tabs q6–8h × 2–3 days
[18]Oxycodone/Acetaminophen (Percocet, Roxicet) 5/325 mg: 1–2 tabs PO	[18]Oxycodone/Acetaminophen (Percocet, Roxicet) 5/325 mg: 1–2 tabs q6–8h × 2–3 days

[1]IBUPROFEN (Motrin, Advil, Nuprin, Rufen, NeoProfen, Caldolor)

▶L ☢ ♀B (D in 3rd trimester) ▶ – ■

ADULT — RA/OA, gout: 200–800 mg PO three to four times per day. Mild to moderate pain: 400 mg PO q4–6h. 400–800 mg IV (Caldolor) q6h prn. 400 mg IV (Caldolor) q4–6h or 100–200 mg q4h prn. Primary dysmenorrhea: 400 mg PO q4h prn. Fever:

200 mg PO q4–6h prn. Migraine pain: 200–400 mg PO not to exceed 400 mg in 24 h unless directed by a physician (OTC dosing). Max dose 3.2 g/day.

PEDS — JRA: 30–50 mg/kg/day PO divided qGh. Max dose 2400 mg/24 h. 20 mg/kg/day may be adequate for milder disease. Analgesic/antipyretic, age older than 6 mo: 5–10 mg/kg PO q6–8h, prn. Max dose 40 mg/kg/day. Patent ductus arteriosus in neonates 32 weeks' gestational age or younger weighing 500–1500 g (NeoProfen): Specialized dosing.

FORMS — OTC: Caps/Liqui-Gel caps 200 mg. Tabs 100, 200 mg. Chewable tabs 100 mg. Susp (infant gtts) 50 mg/1.25 mL (with calibrated dropper), 100 mg/5 mL. Rx Generic/Trade: Tabs 400, 600, 800 mg.

NOTES — May antagonize antiplatelet effects of aspirin if given simultaneously. Take aspirin 2 h prior to ibuprofen. Administer IV (Caldolor) over at least 30 min; hydration important.

MOA — Anti-inflammatory/antipyretic, analgesic.

ADVERSE EFFECTS — Serious: Hypersensitivity, GI bleeding, nephrotoxicity. Frequent: Nausea, dyspepsia.

---

[2]NAPROXEN (Naprosyn, Aleve, Anaprox, EC-Naprosyn, Naprelan, Prevacid, NapraPAC)

▶L ⊗ ♀B (D in 3rd trimester) ▶+ ■

WARNING — Multiple strengths; see FORMS and write specific product on Rx.

ADULT — RA/OA, ankylosing spondylitis, pain, dysmenorrhea, acute tendinitis and bursitis, fever: 250–500 mg PO two times per day. Delayed-release: 375–500 mg PO two times per day (do not crush or chew). Controlled-release: 750–1000 mg PO daily. Acute gout: 750 mg PO once, then 250 mg PO q8h until the attack subsides. Controlled-release: 1000–1500 mg PO once, then 1000 mg PO daily until the attack subsides.

PEDS — JRA: 10–20 mg/kg/day PO divided two times per day (up to 1250 mg/24 h). Pain for age older than 2 yo: 5–7 mg/kg/dose PO q8–12h.

UNAPPROVED ADULT — Acute migraine: 750 mg PO once, then 250–500 mg PO prn. Migraine prophylaxis, menstrual migraine: 500 mg PO two times per day beginning 1 day prior to onset of menses and ending on last day of period.

FORMS — OTC Generic/Trade (Aleve): Tabs, immediate-release 200 mg. OTC Trade only (Aleve): Caps, Gelcaps, immediate-release 200 mg. Rx Generic/Trade: Tabs, immediate-release (Naprosyn) 250, 375, 500 mg. (Anaprox) 275, 550 mg. Tabs, delayed-release enteric-coated (EC-Naprosyn) 375, 500 mg. Tabs, controlled-release (Naprelan) 375, 500, 750 mg. Susp (Naprosyn) 125 mg/5 mL. Prevacid NapraPAC: 7 lansoprazole 15 mg caps packaged with 14 naproxen tabs 375 mg or 500 mg.

NOTES — All dosing is based on naproxen content: 500 mg naproxen is equivalent to 550 mg naproxen sodium.

MOA — Anti-inflammatory, analgesic.

ADVERSE EFFECTS — Serious: Hypersensitivity, GI bleeding, nephrotoxicity. Frequent: Nausea, dyspepsia.

[3]**DICLOFENAC (Voltaren, Voltaren XR, Flector, Zipsor, Cambia, Zorvolex, Voltaren Rapide)**

▶L ⊘ ♀B (D in 3rd trimester) ▶ – $$$ ■

WARNING — Multiple strengths; see FORMS and write specific product on Rx.

ADULT — OA: Immediate- or delayed-release: 50 mg PO two to three times per day or 75 mg two times per day.

Extended-release 100 mg PO daily. Gel: Apply 4 g to knees or 2 g to hands four times per day using enclosed dosing card. RA: Immediate- or delayed-release 50 mg PO three to four times per day or 75 mg two times per day. Extended-release 100 mg PO one to two times per day. Ankylosing spondylitis: Immediate- or delayed-release 25 mg PO four times per day and at bedtime. Analgesia and primary dysmenorrhea: Immediate- or delayed-release 50 mg PO three times per day. Acute pain in strains, sprains, or contusions: Apply 1 patch to painful area two times per day. Acute migraine with or without aura: 50 mg single dose (Cambia), mix packet with 30–60 mL water.

PEDS — Not approved in children.

UNAPPROVED PEDS — JRA: 2–3 mg/kg/day PO.

FORMS — Generic/Trade: Tabs, extended-release (Voltaren XR) 100 mg. Topical gel (Voltaren) 1% 100 g tube. Generic only: Tabs, immediate-release: 25, 50 mg. Generic only: Tabs, delayed-release: 25, 50, 75 mg. Trade only: Patch (Flector) 1.3% diclofenac epolamine. Trade only: Caps, liquid-filled (Zipsor) 25 mg. Caps (Zorvolex) 18, 35 mg. Trade only: Powder for oral soln (Cambia) 50 mg.

NOTES — Check LFTs at baseline, within 4–8 weeks of initiation, then periodically. Do not apply patch to damaged or nonintact skin. Wash hands, and avoid eye contact when handling the patch. Do not wear patch while bathing or showering.

MOA — Anti-inflammatory, analgesic.

ADVERSE EFFECTS — Serious: Hypersensitivity, GI bleeding, hepato/nephrotoxicity. Frequent: Nausea, dyspepsia, pruritus, and dermatitis with patch and gel.

[4]KETOROLAC *(Toradol)*

▶L ✪ ♀B (D in 3rd trimester) ▶ + $$ ◼

WARNING — Indicated for short-term (up to 5 days) therapy only. Ketorolac is a potent NSAID and can cause serious GI and renal adverse effects. It may also increase the risk of bleeding by inhibiting platelet function. Contraindicated in patients with active peptic ulcer disease, recent GI bleeding or perforation, a history of peptic ulcer disease or GI bleeding, or advanced renal impairment.

ADULT — Moderately severe, acute pain, single-dose treatment: 30–60 mg IM or 15–30 mg IV. Multiple-dose treatment: 15–30 mg IV/IM q6h. IV/IM doses are not to exceed 60 mg/day for age 65 yo or older, wt ≤ 50 kg, and patients with moderately elevated serum creatinine. Oral continuation therapy: 1.0 mg PO q4–6h prn, max dose 40 mg/day. Combined duration IV/IM and PO is not to exceed 5 days.

PEDS — Not approved in children.

UNAPPROVED PEDS — Pain: 0.5 mg/kg/dose IM/IV q6h (up to 30 mg q6h or 120 mg/day), give 10 mg PO q6h prn (up to 40 mg/day) for wt > 50 kg.

FORMS — Generic only: Tabs 10 mg.

MOA — Serious: Hypersensitivity, GI bleeding, nephrotoxicity. Frequent: Nausea, dyspepsia.

[5]ACETAMINOPHEN *(Tylenol, Panadol, Tempra, Ofirmev, Paracetamol, Abenol, Atasol, Pediatrix)*

▶LK ♀B ▶+$

ADULT — Analgesic/antipyretic: 325–1000 mg PO q4–6h prn. 650 mg PR q4–6h prn. Max dose 4 g/day. OA: Extended-release: 2 caps PO q8h around the clock. Max dose 6 caps/day.

PEDS – Analgesic/antipyretic: 10–15 mg/kg q4–6h PO/PR prn. Max 5 doses/day.

UNAPPROVED ADULT – OA: 1000 mg PO four times per day.

FORMS – OTC: Tabs 325, 500, 650 mg. Chewable tabs 80 mg. Orally disintegrating tabs 80, 160 mg. Caps/gelcaps 500 mg. Extended-release caplets 650 mg. Liquid 160 mg/ 5 mL, 500 mg/15 mL. Supps 80, 120, 325, 650 mg.

[6]ORAQIX (prilocaine + lidocaine—local anesthetic)

▶LK ♀B ▶? $

ADULT – Local anesthetic gel applied to periodontal pockets using blunt-tipped applicator: 4% injection. The maximum recommended dose of Oraqix at one treatment session is 5 cartridges, i.e., 8.5 g gel. Must be used with special blunt-tipped applicator.

PEDS – Not approved in children.

FORMS – Gel 2.5% + 2.5% with applicator.

NOTES – Do not exceed max dose for lidocaine or prilocaine.

MOA – Amide local anesthetic combination.

ADVERSE EFFECTS – Serious: Seizures, cardiovascular depression, bradycardia, hypersensitivity, methemoglobinemia. Frequent: None.

[7]ARTICAINE (Septocaine, Zorcaine)

▶LK ♀C ▶? $

ADULT – Dental local anesthesia: 4% injection up to 7 mg/ kg total dose.

PEDS – Dental local anesthesia age 4 yo or older: 4% injection up to 7 mg/kg total dose.

FORMS – 4% (includes epinephrine 1:100,000).

NOTES – Do not exceed 7 mg/kg total dose.
MOA – Amide local anesthetic.
ADVERSE EFFECTS – Serious: Seizures, cardiovascular depression, bradycardia, hypersensitivity, methemoglobinemia. Frequent: None.

[8]BUPIVACAINE *(Marcaine, Sensorcaine)*

▶LK ♀C ▶? $ ■
ADULT – Local anesthesia, nerve block: 0.25% injection. Up to 2.5 mg/kg without epinephrine and up 3.0 mg/kg with epinephrine.
PEDS – Not recommended in children younger than 12 yo.
FORMS – 0.25%, 0.5%, 0.75%, all with or without epinephrine.
NOTES – Onset 5 min, duration 2–4 h (longer with epi). Amide group.
MOA – Amide local anesthetic.
ADVERSE EFFECTS – Serious: Seizures, cardiovascular depression, bradycardia, hypersensitivity, methemoglobinemia. Frequent: None.

[9]LIDOCAINE—LOCAL ANESTHETIC *(Xylocaine)*

▶LK ♀B ▶? $
ADULT – Without epinephrine: Max dose 4.5 mg/kg not to exceed 300 mg. With epinephrine: Max dose 7 mg/kg not to exceed 500 mg. Dose for regional block varies by region.
PEDS – Same as adult.
FORMS – 0.5, 1, 1.5, 2%. With epi: 0.5, 1, 1.5, 2%.
NOTES – Onset within 2 min, duration 30–60 min (longer with epi). Amide group. Use "cardiac lidocaine" (ie, IV formulation) for Bier blocks at max dose of 3 mg/kg so that neither epinephrine nor methylparaben is injected IV.

MOA – Amide local anesthetic.
ADVERSE EFFECTS – Serious: Seizures, cardiovascular depression, bradycardia, hypersensitivity, methemoglobinemia. Frequent: None.

[10]MEPIVACAINE *(Carbocaine, Polocaine)*

▶LK ♀C ▶? $

ADULT – Nerve block: 1–2% injection. Onset 3–5 min, duration 45–90 min. Amide group. Max local dose 5–6 mg/kg.
PEDS – Nerve block: 1–2% injection. Use less than 2% concentration if age younger than 3 yo or wt < 30 pounds. Max local dose 5–6 mg/kg.
FORMS – 1, 1.5, 2, 3%.
NOTES – Onset 3–5 min, duration 45–90 min. Amide group. Max local dose 5–6 mg/kg.
MOA – Amide local anesthetic.
ADVERSE EFFECTS – Serious: Seizures, cardiovascular depression, bradycardia, hypersensitivity, methemoglobinemia, nephrotoxicity. Frequent: None.

[11]PRILOCAINE *(Citanest)*

▶LK ♀B ▶? $

ADULT – Nerve block and dental procedures: 4% injection. Maximum local dose is 5 mg/kg without epinephrine and 7 mg/kg with epinephrine.
PEDS – Nerve block and dental procedures, age older than 9 mo: 4% injection. If younger than 5 yo, maximum local dose is 3–4 mg/kg (with or without epinephrine). If 5 yo or older, maximum local dose is 5 mg/kg without epinephrine and 7 mg/kg with epinephrine.

FORMS – 4%, 4% with epinephrine.
NOTES – Contraindicated if younger than 6–9 mo. If younger than 5 yo, max local dose is 3–4 mg/kg (with or without epinephrine). If 5 yo or older, max local dose is 5 mg/kg without epinephrine and 7 mg/kg with epinephrine.
MOA – Amide local anesthetic.
ADVERSE EFFECTS – Serious: Seizures, cardiovascular depression, bradycardia, hypersensitivity, methemoglobinemia. Frequent: None.

[12]PROCAINE *(Novocain)*

▶Plasma ♀C ▶? $
ADULT – Local and regional anesthesia: 1–2% injection. Spinal anesthesia: 10%.
PEDS – Local and regional anesthesia: 1–2% injection. Spinal anesthesia: 10%.
FORMS – 1, 2, 10%.
NOTES – Trade name is included only for reference; Novocain brand was discontinued.
MOA – Ester local anesthetic.
ADVERSE EFFECTS – Serious: Seizures, cardiovascular depression, bradycardia, hypersensitivity, methemoglobinemia. Frequent: None.

[13]ROPIVACAINE *(Naropin)*

▶LK ♀B ▶? $
WARNING – Inadvertent intravascular injection may result in arrhythmia or cardiac arrest.
ADULT – Local and regional anesthesia: 0.2–1% injection.
PEDS – Not approved in children.

FORMS – 0.2, 0.5, 0.75, 1%.

MOA – Amide local anesthetic.

ADVERSE EFFECTS – Serious: Seizures, cardiovascular depression, bradycardia, hypersensitivity, methemoglobinemia. Frequent: None.

[14]**MORPHINE** *(MS Contin, Kadian, Avinza, Roxanol, Oramorph SR, MSIR, DepoDur, Statex, M.O.S. Doloral, M-Eslon)*

▶L ♀C ▶? ©III $■

WARNING – Multiple strengths; see FORMS and write specific product on Rx. Drinking alcohol while taking Avinza may result in a rapid release of a potentially fatal dose of morphine.

ADULT – Moderate to severe pain: 10–30 mg PO q4h (immediate-release tabs, or oral soln). Controlled-release (MS Contin, Oramorph SR): 30 mg PO q8–12h. (Kadian): 20 mg PO q12–24h. Extended-release caps (Avinza): 30 mg PO daily. 10 mg q4h IM/SC. 2.5–15 mg/70 kg IV over 4–5 min. 10–20 mg PR q4h. Pain with major surgery (DepoDur): 10–15 mg once epidurally at the lumbar level prior to surgery (max dose 20 mg), or 10 mg epidurally after clamping of the umbilical cord with cesarean section.

PEDS – Moderate to severe pain: 0.1–0.2 mg/kg up to 15 mg IM/SC/IV q2–4h.

UNAPPROVED PEDS – Moderate to severe pain: 0.2–0.5 mg/kg/dose PO (immediate-release) q4–6h; 0.3–0.6 mg/kg/dose PO (controlled-release) q12h.

FORMS – Generic only: Tabs, immediate-release 15, 30 mg ($). Oral soln 10 mg/5 mL, 20 mg/5 mL, 20 mg/mL (concentrate). Rectal supps 5, 10, 20, 30 mg. Generic/Trade: Controlled-release tabs (MS Contin) 15, 30, 60, 100, 200 mg ($$$$). Controlled-release caps (Kadian) 10, 20, 30, 50, 60, 80, 100 mg ($$$$$). Extended-release caps (Avinza) 30, 45, 60, 75, 90, 120 mg. Trade only: Controlled-release caps (Kadian) 40, 200 mg.

NOTES – Titrate dose as high as necessary to relieve cancer or nonmalignant pain where chronic opioids are necessary. The active metabolites may accumulate in hepatic/renal insufficiency and the elderly leading to increased analgesic and sedative effects. Do not break, chew, or crush MS Contin or Oramorph SR. Kadian and Avinza caps may be opened and sprinkled in applesauce for easier administration; however, the pellets should not be crushed or chewed. Doses more than 1600 mg/day of Avinza contain a potentially nephrotoxic quantity of fumaric acid. Do not mix DepoDur with other medications; do not administer any other medications into epidural space for at least 48 h. Severe opiate overdose with respiratory depression has occurred with intrathecal leakage of DepoDur.

MOA – Opioid agonist analgesic.

ADVERSE EFFECTS – Serious: Respiratory depression/arrest. Frequent: N/V, constipation, sedation, hypotension.

[15]NORCO *(hydrocodone + acetaminophen)*

▶L ✪ ♀C ▶? ⊙II $$

WARNING – Multiple strengths; see FORMS and write specific product on Rx.

ADULT – Moderate to severe pain: 1–2 tabs PO q4–6h prn (5/325), max dose 12 tabs/day. 1 tab (7.5/325 and 10/325) PO q4–6h prn, max dose 8 and 6 tabs/day, respectively.

PEDS – Not approved in children.

FORMS – Generic/Trade: Tabs 5/325, 7.5/325, 10/325 mg hydrocodone/acetaminophen, scored. Generic only: Soln 7.5/325 mg per 15 mL.

[16]VICODIN *(hydrocodone + acetaminophen)*

▶LK ✪ ♀C ? ⊙II $$$

WARNING – Multiple strengths; see FORMS and write specific product on Rx.

ADULT – Moderate pain: 5/300 mg (max dose 8 tabs/day) and 7.5/300 mg (max dose of 6 tabs/day): 1–2 tabs PO q4–6h prn. 10/300 mg: 1 tab PO q4–6h prn (max of 6 tabs/day).

PEDS – Not approved in children.

FORMS – Generic/Trade: Tabs Vicodin (5/300), Vicodin ES (7.5/300), Vicodin HP (10/300) mg hydrocodone/mg acetaminophen, scored.

[16]LORTAB *(hydrocodone + acetaminophen)*

▶LK ✪ ♀C ▶ ⊙II $$

WARNING – Multiple strengths; see FORMS and write specific product on Rx.

ADULT – Moderate pain: 1–2 tabs 2.5/325 and 5/325 PO q4–6h prn, max dose 8 tabs/day. 1 tab 7.5/325 and 10/325 PO q4–6h prn, max dose 5 tabs/day.

PEDS – Not approved in children.

FORMS – Generic/Trade: Lortab 5/325 (scored), Lortab 7.5/325 (trade scored), Lortab 10/325 mg hydrocodone/mg acetaminophen. Generic only: Tabs 2.5/325 mg.

MOA – Serious: Respiratory depression/arrest, hepatotoxicity. Frequent: N/V, constipation, sedation.

[16]LORCET (hydrocodone + acetaminophen)

▶LK ☻♀–▶? ©II $$
WARNING – Multiple strengths; see FORMS and write specific product on Rx.
ADULT – Moderate pain: 1–2 caps (5/325) PO q4–6h prn, max dose 8 caps/day. 1 tab PO q4–6h prn (7.5/325 and 10/325), max dose 6 tabs/day.
PEDS – Not approved in children.
FORMS – Generic/Trade: Tabs, 5/325, 7.5/325,10/325 mg.

[17]VICOPROFEN (hydrocodone + ibuprofen)

▶LK ☻♀–▶? ©II $$
ADULT – Moderate pain: 1 tab PO q4–6h prn, max dose 5 tabs/day.
PEDS – Not approved in children.
FORMS – Generic only: Tabs 2.5/200, 5/200,7.5/200, 10/200 mg hydrocodone/ibuprofen.
NOTES – See NSAIDs: Other subclass warning.
MOA – Combination analgesic.
ADVERSE EFFECTS – Serious: Respiratory depression/arrest, hypersensitivity, GI bleeding, nephrotoxicity. Frequent: N/V, constipation, dyspepsia, sedation.

[18]PERCOCET (oxycodone + acetaminophen, Percocet-Demi, Oxycocet, Endocet)

▶L ☻♀C▶– ©II $
WARNING – Multiple strengths; see FORMS and write specific product on Rx.

ADULT — Moderate to severe pain: 1–2 tabs PO q4–6h prn (2.5/325 and 5/325 mg). 1 tab PO q4–6h prn (7.5/325 and 10/325 mg).

PEDS — Not approved in children.

FORMS — Generic/Trade: Oxycodone/acetaminophen tabs 2.5/325, 5/325, 7.5/325, 10/325 mg. Trade only: (Primlev) tabs 2.5/300, 5/300, 7.5/300, 10/300 mg. Generic only: 10/325 mg.

[18]ROXICET *(oxycodone + acetaminophen)*

▶L ⊗ ♀C ▶– ©II $

WARNING — Multiple strengths; see FORMS and write specific product on Rx.

ADULT — Moderate to severe pain: 1 tab PO q6h prn. Oral soln: 5 mL PO q6h prn.

PEDS — Not approved in children.

FORMS — Generic/Trade: Tabs 5/325 mg. Caps/caplets 5/325 mg. Soln 5/325 per 5 mL mg oxycodone/acetaminophen.

HEADACHE

Inpatient Analgesics (in the ED)	Outpatient Analgesics (discharge)
Non-Opioid	**Non-Opioid**
<u>Oral/Intranasal Regimen:</u> [1]**Acetaminophen/Aspirin/Caffeine (Excedrin):** 1–2 caplets [2]**Ibuprofen:** 400 mg, or [3]**Naproxen:** 500 mg, or [4]**Diclofenac:** 50 mg, or [5]**Ketorolac:** 10 mg [6]**Acetaminophen:** 500 mg q8h (max 1500 mg/day). Best if combined with [2]**Ibuprofen** at 400 mg q8h. [7]**Sumatriptan:** 100 mg [7]**Intranasal (IN) Sumatriptan:** 5–20 mg dose, repeat after 2h <u>Regional Anesthesia and Analgesia (Cervicogenic Headache, Migraine Headache, Tension Headache: Greater/Lesser Occipital Nerve Block):</u> [8]**Articane:** 4%, max 7 mg/kg [9]**Bupivacaine** w/o epi: 0.25–0.5%, max 2.5 mg/kg	[26]**Aspirin:** 325–650 mg q6h [1]**Acetaminophen/Aspirin/Caffeine (Excedrin):** 2 caplets q6–8h × 2–3 days [2]**PO Ibuprofen:** 400 mg q8h × 3 days (max 5 days with 1200 mg/d) [3]**PO Naproxen:** 500 mg q12h × 3 days (max 5 days) [6]**PO Acetaminophen:** 500 mg PO q8h (max 1500 mg/day). Best if combined with [2]**Ibuprofen** at 400 mg q8h. [7]**PO Sumatriptan:** 100 mg (no more than 200 mg per 24 h) [7]**Intranasal (IN) Sumatriptan:** 5–20 mg, repeat after 2h, max 40 mg daily

(continues)

Inpatient Analgesics (in the ED)	Outpatient Analgesics (discharge)
Non-Opioid	**Non-Opioid**
[9]**Bupivacaine** with epi: 0.25–0.5%, max 3.0 mg/kg	[27]**PO Rizatriptan:** 10 mg (no more than 20 mg per 24 h)
[10]**Lidocaine** w/o epi: 0.5–2%, 4.5 mg/kg, max 300 mg	
[10]**Lidocaine** with epi: 0.5–2%, 7 mg/kg, max 500 mg	
[11]**Mepivacaine:** 1–2%, max 5 mg/kg	
[12]**Prilocaine:** 4%, max 5 mg/kg w/o epi, 7 mg/kg with epi	
[13]**Procaine:** 0.25–0.5%, max 6 mg/kg	
[14]**Ropivacaine:** 0.2–1%, max 3 mg/kg	
[15]**Chloroprocaine:** 2–3%, max 11 mg/kg	
Paracervical Block (Intramuscular Injection):	
[8]**Articane:** 4% max 7 mg/kg	
[9]**Bupivacaine** w/o epi: 0.25–0.5%, max 2.5 mg/kg	
[9]**Bupivacaine** with epi: 0.25–0.5%, max 3.0 mg/kg	
[10]**Lidocaine** w/o epi: 0.5–2%, 4.5 mg/kg, max 300 mg	

(continues)

Inpatient Analgesics (in the ED)	Outpatient Analgesics (discharge)
Non-Opioid	**Non-Opioid**
[10]**Lidocaine** with epi: 0.5–2%, 7 mg/kg, max 500 mg	
[11]**Mepivacaine:** 1–2%, max 5 mg/kg	
[12]**Prilocaine:** 4%, max 5 mg/kg w/o epi, 7 mg/kg with epi	
[13]**Procaine:** 0.25–0.5%, max 6 mg/kg	
[14]**Ropivacaine:** 0.2–1%, max 3 mg/kg	
[15]**Chloroprocaine:** 2–3%, max 11 mg/kg	
<u>Parenteral Regimen:</u>	
[16]**IV Metoclopramide:** 10 mg (slow infusion over 10–15 min), can be repeated in 1–2 h	
[17]**IV Prochlorperazine:** 10 mg (slow infusion over 10–15 min) with [18]**IV Diphenhydramine:** 25–50 mg (for akathisia/ agitation prophylaxis), can be repeated in 1–2 h	
[19]**IV Chlorpromazine:** 12.5 mg (slow infusion in 500 mL over 30 min)	

(continues)

Inpatient Analgesics (in the ED)	Outpatient Analgesics (discharge)
Non-Opioid	**Non-Opioid**
[5]**IV Ketorolac:** 10–15 mg	
[20]**IV Magnesium:** 1–2 gm over 30–60 min	
[21]**IV Valproate Sodium:** 500–1000 mg IV over 60 min, may repeat in 2h	
[22]**IV Dexamethasone:** 10 mg IV (decreases migraine recurrence)	
[7]**SQ Sumatriptan (migraine):** 6 mg (within 1 hr of onset, 12 mg 1hr later if needed)	
Refractory cases:	
[23]**IV Haldol:** 2.5–5 mg IV (slow infusion over 15–30 min)	
[24]**IV Propofol (intractable migraine):** 10 mg IVP q5 min until HA is tolerable (max dose 100 mg)	
[25]**Ketamine (Subdissociative Dose, SDK)** • **IV:** 0.3 mg/kg over 15 min, +/− continuous IV infusion at 0.15–0.2 mg/kg/h • **SQ:** 0.3 mg/kg over 15 min, +/− continuous SQ infusion at 0.15–0.2 mg/kg/h	

[1]EXCEDRIN MIGRAINE *(acetaminophen + acetylsalicylic acid + caffeine)*

▶LK ♀D ▶? $

ADULT – Migraine headache: 2 tabs/caps/geltabs PO q6h while symptoms persist. Max 8 tabs in 24 h.

PEDS – Use adult dose for age 12 or older.

FORMS – OTC Generic/Trade: Tabs/caps/geltabs 250 mg acetaminophen/250 mg aspirin/65 mg caffeine.

NOTES – See NSAIDs: Salicylic acid subclass warning. Avoid concomitant use of other acetaminophen-containing products.

MOA – Combination analgesic.

ADVERSE EFFECTS – Serious: Hepatotoxicity, hypersensitivity, Reye's syndrome, GI bleeding, nephrotoxicity. Frequent: Dyspepsia, nervousness, insomnia.

[2]IBUPROFEN *(Motrin, Advil, Nuprin, Rufen, NeoProfen, Caldolor)*

▶L ⊗ ♀B (D in 3rd trimester) ▶+ ■

ADULT – RA/OA, gout: 200–800 mg PO three to four times per day. Mild to moderate pain: 400 mg PO q4–6h. 400–800 mg IV (Caldolor) q6h prn. 400 mg IV (Caldolor) q4–6h or 100–200 mg q4h prn. Primary dysmenorrhea: 400 mg PO q4h prn. Fever: 200 mg PO q4–6h prn. Migraine pain: 200–400 mg PO not to exceed 400 mg in 24 h unless directed by a physician (OTC dosing). Max dose 3.2 g/day.

PEDS – JRA: 30–50 mg/kg/day PO divided qGh. Max dose 2400 mg/24 h. 20 mg/kg/day may be adequate for milder disease. Analgesic/antipyretic, age older than 6 mo: 5–10 mg/kg PO q6–8h prn. Max dose 40 mg/kg/day. Patent ductus arteriosus

HEADACHE

in neonates 32 weeks' gestational age or younger weighing 500–1500 g (NeoProfen): Specialized dosing.

FORMS – OTC: Caps/Liqui-Gel caps 200 mg. Tabs 100, 200 mg. Chewable tabs 100 mg. Susp (infant gtts) 50 mg/1.25 mL (with calibrated dropper), 100 mg/5 mL. Rx Generic/Trade: Tabs 400, 600, 800 mg.

NOTES – May antagonize antiplatelet effects of aspirin if given simultaneously. Take aspirin 2 h prior to ibuprofen. Administer IV (Caldolor) over at least 30 min; hydration important.

MOA – Anti-inflammatory/antipyretic, analgesic.

ADVERSE EFFECTS – Serious: Hypersensitivity, GI bleeding, nephrotoxicity. Frequent: Nausea, dyspepsia.

[3]NAPROXEN (Naprosyn, Aleve, Anaprox, EC-Naprosyn, Naprelan, Prevacid, NapraPAC)

▶L ⊗ ♀B (D in 3rd trimester) ▶+ $■

WARNING – Multiple strengths; see FORMS and write specific product on Rx.

ADULT – RA/OA, ankylosing spondylitis, pain, dysmenorrhea, acute tendinitis and bursitis, fever: 250–500 mg PO two times per day. Delayed-release: 375–500 mg PO two times per day (do not crush or chew). Controlled-release: 750–1000 mg PO daily. Acute gout: 750 mg PO once, then 250 mg PO q8h until the attack subsides. Controlled-release: 1000–1500 mg PO once, then 1000 mg PO daily until the attack subsides.

PEDS – JRA: 10–20 mg/kg/day PO divided two times per day (up to 1250 mg/24 h). Pain for age older than 2 yo: 5–7 mg/kg/dose PO q8–12h.

UNAPPROVED ADULT – Acute migraine: 750 mg PO once, then 250–500 mg PO prn. Migraine prophylaxis, menstrual migraine:

500 mg PO two times per day beginning 1 day prior to onset of menses and ending on last day of period.

FORMS – OTC Generic/Trade (Aleve): Tabs, immediate-release 200 mg. OTC Trade only (Aleve): Caps, gelcaps, immediate-release 200 mg. Rx Generic/Trade: Tabs, immediate-release (Naprosyn) 250, 375, 500 mg. (Anaprox) 275, 550 mg. Tabs, delayed-release enteric-coated (EC-Naprosyn) 375, 500 mg. Tabs, controlled-release (Naprelan) 375, 500, 750 mg. Susp (Naprosyn) 125 mg/5 mL. Prevacid NapraPAC: 7 lansoprazole 15 mg caps packaged with 14 naproxen tabs 375 mg or 500 mg.

NOTES – All dosing is based on naproxen content: 500 mg naproxen is equivalent to 550 mg naproxen sodium.

MOA – Anti-inflammatory, analgesic.

ADVERSE EFFECTS – Serious: Hypersensitivity, GI bleeding, nephrotoxicity. Frequent: Nausea, dyspepsia.

[4]DICLOFENAC *(Voltaren, Voltaren XR, Flector, Zipsor, Cambia, Zorvolex, Voltaren Rapide)*

▶L ⊗ ♀B (D in 3rd trimester) ▶– $$$ ■

WARNING – Multiple strengths; see FORMS and write specific product on Rx.

ADULT – OA: Immediate- or delayed-release: 50 mg PO two to three times per day or 75 mg two times per day. Extended-release 100 mg PO daily. Gel: Apply 4 g to knees or 2 g to hands four times per day using enclosed dosing card. RA: Immediate- or delayed-release 50 mg PO three to four times per day or 75 mg two times per day. Extended-release 100 mg PO one to two times per day. Ankylosing spondylitis: Immediate- or delayed-release 25 mg PO four times per day and at bedtime. Analgesia and primary dysmenorrhea:

Immediate- or delayed-release 50 mg PO three times per day. Acute pain in strains, sprains, or contusions: Apply 1 patch to painful area two times per day. Acute migraine with or without aura: 50 mg single dose (Cambia), mix packet with 30–60 mL water.

PEDS — Not approved in children.

UNAPPROVED PEDS — JRA: 2–3 mg/kg/day PO.

FORMS — Generic/Trade: Tabs, extended-release (Voltaren XR) 100 mg. Topical gel (Voltaren) 1% 100 g tube. Generic only: Tabs, immediate-release: 25, 50 mg. Generic only: Tabs, delayed-release: 25, 50, 75 mg. Trade only: Patch (Flector) 1.3% diclofenac epolamine. Trade only: Caps, liquid-filled (Zipsor) 25 mg. Caps (Zorvolex) 18, 35 mg. Trade only: Powder for oral soln (Cambia) 50 mg.

NOTES — Check LFTs at baseline, within 4–8 weeks of initiation, then periodically. Do not apply patch to damaged or nonintact skin. Wash hands, and avoid eye contact when handling the patch. Do not wear patch while bathing or showering.

MOA — Anti-inflammatory, analgesic.

ADVERSE EFFECTS — Serious: Hypersensitivity, GI bleeding, hepato/nephrotoxicity. Frequent: Nausea, dyspepsia, pruritus, and dermatitis with patch and gel.

[5]KETOROLAC (Toradol)

▶L ⊗ ♀B (D in 3rd trimester) ▶+ $$■

WARNING — Indicated for short-term (up to 5 days) therapy only. Ketorolac is a potent NSAID and can cause serious GI and renal adverse effects. It may also increase the risk of bleeding by inhibiting platelet function. Contraindicated in patients with active peptic ulcer disease, recent GI bleeding or perforation, a history of peptic ulcer disease or GI bleeding, or advanced renal impairment.

ADULT — Moderately severe, acute pain, single-dose treatment: 30–60 mg IM or 15–30 mg IV. Multiple-dose treatment: 15–30 mg IV/IM q6h. IV/IM doses are not to exceed 60 mg/day for age 65 yo or older, wt > 50 kg, and patients with moderately elevated serum creatinine. Oral continuation therapy: 1.0 mg PO q4–6h prn, max dose 40 mg/day. Combined duration IV/IM and PO is not to exceed 5 days.

PEDS — Not approved in children.

UNAPPROVED PEDS — Pain: 0.5 mg/kg/dose IM/IV q6h (up to 30 mg q6h or 120 mg/day), give 10 mg PO q6h pm (up to 40 mg/day) for wt > 50 kg.

FORMS — Generic only: Tabs 10 mg.

MOA — Serious: Hypersensitivity, GI bleeding, nephrotoxicity. Frequent: Nausea, dyspepsia.

[6]ACETAMINOPHEN (Tylenol, Panadol, Tempra, Ofirmev, Paracetamol, Abenol, Atasol, Pediatrix)

▶LK ♀B ▶+ $

ADULT — Analgesic/antipyretic: 325–1000 mg PO q4–6h pm. 650 mg PR q4–6h pm. Max dose 4 g/day. OA: Extended-release: 2 caps PO q8h around the clock. Max dose 6 caps/day.

PEDS — Analgesic/antipyretic: 10–15 mg/kg q4–6h PO/PR pm. Max 5 doses/day.

UNAPPROVED ADULT — OA: 1000 mg PO four times per day.

FORMS — OTC: Tabs 325, 500, 650 mg. Chewable tabs 80 mg. Orally disintegrating tabs 80, 160 mg. Caps/gelcaps 500 mg. Extended-release caplets 650 mg. Liquid 160 mg/5 mL, 500 mg/15 mL. Supps 80, 120, 325, 650 mg.

[7]SUMATRIPTAN (Zembrace SymTouch, Onzetra Xsail, Imitrex, Alsuma, Sumavel, Zecuity)

▶LK ♀C Embryotoxicity reported in animals. Registry available. ▶+ $

ADULT — Migraine Treatment: Imitrex: 1–6 mg (6 mg usual) SC. May repeat in 1 h prn if there was some response to first dose. Max 12 mg/24 h. If HA returns after initial SC injection, then single tabs may be used q2h prn, max 100 mg/24 h. Zembrace SymTouch: 3 mg SC. May repeat after 1 h or longer prn up to three times or max of 12 mg/24 h. Tabs: 25–100 mg PO (50 mg most common). May repeat q2h prn with 25–100 mg doses. Max 200 mg/24 h. Initial oral dose of 50 mg appears to be more effective than 25 mg. Intranasal spray: 5–20 mg q2h. Max 40 mg/24 h. Intranasal powder: 22 mg (11 mg in each nostril). May repeat if needed at least 2 h after the first dose. Max 44 mg/24 h. Transdermal (Zecuity): 1 patch topically, max two patches/24 h with no less than 2 h before second application. No evidence of increased benefit with second patch. Cluster headache treatment: 6 mg SC. May repeat after 1 h or longer prn if there was some response to first dose. Max 12 mg/24 h. Avoid MAOIs.

PEDS — Not approved in children.

UNAPPROVED PEDS — Acute migraine, intranasal spray, for age 8–17 yo: Give 20 mg for wt 40 kg or greater or 10 mg for wt 20–39 kg intranasally at headache onset. May repeat after 2 h prn.

FORMS — Generic/Trade: Tabs 25, 50, 100 mg. Injection (STATdose System) 4-, 6-mg prefilled cartridges. Trade only: Nasal spray (Imitrex Nasal) 5, 20 mg (box of #6). Alsuma, Sumavel: Injection 6-mg prefilled cartridge. Injection (Zembrace SymTouch)

3-mg autoinjector. Zecuity Transdermal Patch (temporarily suspended, June 2016): 6.5 mg/4 h. Generic only: Nasal spray 5, 20 mg (box of #6). Intranasal powder: 11 mg/nosepiece.

NOTES – Should not be combined with MAOIs. Do not use with ergots. Avoid IM/IV route. The Zecuity patch is a battery-powered iontophoretic system. The FDA reported in 2016 that some patients have reported burns and scarring at application sites with this patch. Patients reporting moderate to severe pain at the site should remove the patch immediately and contact their healthcare professional. Do not bathe, swim, or shower while wearing the patch. The product was temporarily suspended in June, 2016.

MOA – Serotonin 5-HT1B/D agonist.

ADVERSE EFFECTS – Serious: Chest pain/tightness, coronary vasospasm, acute MI, arrhythmias, peripheral ischemia, stroke, seizures, HTN, medication overuse headache, serotonin syndrome. Frequent: Dizziness, lightheadedness, weakness, myalgias, muscle cramps, N/V, fatigue, drowsiness, flushing, pain/pressure sensation.

[8]ARTICAINE *(Septocaine, Zorcaine)*

▶LK ♀C ▶? $

ADULT – Dental local anesthesia: 4% injection up to 7 mg/kg total dose.

PEDS – Dental local anesthesia: age 4 yo or older: 4% injection up to 7 mg/kg total dose.

FORMS – 4% (includes epinephrine 1:100,000).

NOTES – Do not exceed 7 mg/kg total dose.

MOA – Amide local anesthetic.

[9]BUPIVACAINE *(Marcaine, Sensorcaine)*

▶LK ♀C ▶? $ ■

ADULT – Local anesthesia, nerve block: 0.25% injection. Up to 2.5 mg/kg without epinephrine and up 3.0 mg/kg with epinephrine.

PEDS – Not recommended in children younger than 12 yo.

FORMS – 0.25%, 0.5%, 0.75%, all with or without epinephrine.

NOTES – Onset 5 min, duration 2–4 h (longer with epi). Amide group.

MOA – Amide local anesthetic.

ADVERSE EFFECTS – Serious: Seizures, cardiovascular depression, bradycardia, hypersensitivity, methemoglobinemia. Frequent: None.

[10]LIDOCAINE—LOCAL ANESTHETIC *(Xylocaine)*

▶LK ♀B ▶? $

ADULT – Without epinephrine: Max dose 4.5 mg/kg not to exceed 300 mg. With epinephrine: Max dose 7 mg/kg not to exceed 500 mg. Dose for regional block varies by region.

PEDS – Same as adult.

FORMS – 0.5, 1, 1.5, 2%. With epi: 0.5, 1, 1.5, 2%.

NOTES – Onset within 2 min, duration 30–60 min (longer with epi). Amide group. Use "cardiac lidocaine" (ie, IV formulation) for Bier blocks at max dose of 3 mg/kg so that neither epinephrine nor methylparaben is injected IV.

MOA – Amide local anesthetic.

ADVERSE EFFECTS – Serious: Seizures, cardiovascular depression, bradycardia, hypersensitivity, methemoglobinemia. Frequent: None.

¹¹ MEPIVACAINE *(Carbocaine, Polocaine)*

▶LK ♀C ▶? $

ADULT – Nerve block: 1–2% injection. Onset 3–5 min, duration 45 to 90 min. Amide group. Max local dose 5–6 mg/kg.

PEDS – Nerve block: 1–2% injection. Use less than 2% concentration if age younger than 3 yo or wt < 30 pounds. Max local dose 5–6 mg/kg.

FORMS – 1, 1.5, 2, 3%.

NOTES – Onset 3–5 min, duration 45–90 min. Amide group. Max local dose 5–6 mg/kg.

MOA – Amide local anesthetic.

ADVERSE EFFECTS – Serious: Seizures, cardiovascular depression, bradycardia, hypersensitivity, methemoglobinemia, nephrotoxicity. Frequent: None.

¹²PRILOCAINE *(Citanest)*

▶LK ♀B ▶? $

ADULT – Nerve block and dental procedures: 4% injection. Maximum local dose is 5 mg/kg without epinephrine and 7 mg/kg with epinephrine.

PEDS – Nerve block and dental procedures, age older than 9 mo: 4% injection. If younger than 5 yo, maximum local dose is 3–4 mg/kg (with or without epinephrine). If 5 yo or older, maximum local dose is 5 mg/kg without epinephrine and 7 mg/kg with epinephrine.

FORMS – 4%, 4% with epinephrine.

NOTES – Contraindicated if younger than 6–9 mo. If younger than 5 yo, max local dose is 3–4 mg/kg (with or without epinephrine). If 5 yo or older, max local dose is 5 mg/kg without epinephrine and 7 mg/kg with epinephrine.

MOA – Amide local anesthetic.
ADVERSE EFFECTS – Serious: Seizures, cardiovascular depression, bradycardia, hypersensitivity, methemoglobinemia. Frequent: None.

[13]PROCAINE *(Novocain)*

▶Plasma ♀C ▶? $
ADULT – Local and regional anesthesia: 1–2% injection. Spinal anesthesia: 10%.
PEDS – Local and regional anesthesia: 1–2% injection. Spinal anesthesia: 10%.
FORMS – 1, 2, 10%.
NOTES – Trade name is included only for reference; Novocain brand was discontinued.
MOA – Ester local anesthetic.
ADVERSE EFFECTS – Serious: Seizures, cardiovascular depression, bradycardia, hypersensitivity, methemoglobinemia. Frequent: None.

[14]ROPIVACAINE *(Naropin)*

▶LK ♀B ▶? $
WARNING – Inadvertent intravascular injection may result in arrhythmia or cardiac arrest.
ADULT – Local and regional anesthesia: 0.2–1% injection.
PEDS – Not approved in children.
FORMS – 0.2, 0.5, 0.75, 1%.
MOA – Amide local anesthetic.
ADVERSE EFFECTS – Serious: Seizures, cardiovascular depression, bradycardia, hypersensitivity, methemoglobinemia. Frequent: None.

[15]CHLOROPROCAINE (Nesacaine)

▶LK ♀C ▷? $

ADULT – Epidural anesthesia: 18–24 mL of 2.0–3.0% chloroprocaine will provide 30–60 min of surgical anesthesia. Infiltration and peripheral nerve block: 0.5–40 mL of 1–3% chloroprocaine.

PEDS – Same as adult, age 3 yo or older.

FORMS – 1, 2, 3%.

NOTES – Max local dose: 11 mg/kg.

MOA – Ester local anesthetic.

ADVERSE EFFECTS – Serious: Seizures, cardiovascular depression, bradycardia, hypersensitivity, methemoglobinemia. Frequent: None.

[16]METOCLOPRAMIDE (Reglan, Metozolv ODT, Maxeran)

▶K ⊗ ♀B ▷? $

WARNING – Irreversible tardive dyskinesia with high dose or long-term (greater than 3 mon) use.

ADULT – GERD: 10–15 mg PO four times per day 30 min before meals and at bedtime. Diabetic gastroparesis: 10 mg PO/IV/IM 30 min before meals and at bedtime. Prevention of chemo-induced emesis: 1–2 mg/kg PO/IV/IM 30 min before chemo then q2h for 2 doses then q3h for 3 doses prn. Prevention of post-op nausea: 10–20 mg IM/IV near end of surgical procedure, may repeat q3–4h prn. Intubation of small intestine: 10 mg IV. Radiographic exam of upper GI tract: 10 mg IV.

PEDS – Intubation of small intestine: 0.1 mg/kg IV for age younger than 6 yo; 2.5–5 mg IV for age 6–14 yo. Radiographic exam of upper GI tract: 0.1 mg/kg IV for age younger than 6 yo; 2.5–5 mg IV for age 6–14 yo.

HEADACHE

UNAPPROVED ADULT — Prevention/treatment of chemo-induced emesis: 3 mg/kg IV over 1 h followed by continuous IV infusion of 0.5 mg/kg/h for 12 h. Migraine treatment: 10 mg IV. Migraine adjunct: 10 mg PO 5–10 min before ergotamine/analgesic/sedative.

UNAPPROVED PEDS — Gastroesophageal reflux: 0.4–0.8 mg/kg/day in 4 divided doses. Prevention of chemo-induced emesis: 1–2 mg/kg 30 min before chemo and then q3h prn (up to 5 doses/day or 5–10 mg/kg/day).

FORMS — Generic/Trade: Tabs 5, 10 mg. Orally disintegrating tabs 5, 10 mg (Metozolv). Generic only: Oral soln 5 mg/5 mL.

NOTES — To reduce incidence and severity of akathisia, consider giving IV doses over 15 min. If extrapyramidal reactions occur (especially with high IV doses) give diphenhydramine IM/IV. Adjust dose in renal dysfunction. Irreversible tardive dyskinesia with high dose or long-term (greater than 12 weeks) use. Avoid use greater than 12 weeks except in rare cases where benefit outweighs risk of tardive dyskinesia. May cause drowsiness, agitation, seizures, hallucinations, galactorrhea, hyperprolactinemia, constipation, diarrhea. Increases cyclosporine and ethanol absorption. Do not use if bowel perforation or mechanical obstruction present. Levodopa decreases metoclopramide effects.

MOA — Dopamine blockade; inhibits chemoreceptor trigger zone.

ADVERSE EFFECTS — Frequent: Restlessness, drowsiness, diarrhea, asthenia.

[17]PROCHLORPERAZINE (Compazine, Stemetil)

▶LK ♀C ▶? $

ADULT — N/V: 5–10 mg PO/IM three to four times per day (up to 40 mg/day). Sustained release: 10 mg PO q12h or 15 mg q AM.

Suppository: 25 mg PR q12h. IV/IM: 5–10 mg IV over at least 2 min q3–4h prn (up to 40 mg/day); 5–10 mg IM q3–4h prn (up to 40 mg/day).

PEDS – N/V: Not recommended in age younger than 2 yo or wt < 10 kg, 0.4 mg/kg/day PO/PR in 3–4 divided doses for age older than 2 yo; 0.1–0.15 mg/kg/dose IM; IV not recommended in children.

UNAPPROVED ADULT – Migraine: 10 mg IV/IM or 25 mg PR single dose for acute headache.

UNAPPROVED PEDS – N/V during surgery: 5–10 mg IM 1–2 h before anesthesia induction, may repeat in 30 min; 5–10 mg IV 15–30 min before anesthesia induction, may repeat once.

FORMS – Generic only: Tabs 5, 10, 25 mg. Generic/Trade: Supp 25 mg.

NOTES – May cause extrapyramidal reactions (especially in elderly), hypotension (with IV) arrhythmias, sedation, seizures, hyperprolactinemia, gynecomastia, dry mouth, constipation, urinary retention, leukopenia, thrombocytopenia. Elderly more prone to adverse effects. Brand name Compazine no longer available.

MOA – Blocks post-synaptic dopaminergic receptors.

ADVERSE EFFECTS – Frequent: None. Severe: Cardiac arrest, hypotension, extrapyramidal signs.

HEADACHE

---

[18]**DIPHENHYDRAMINE** *(Benadryl, Banophen, AllerMax, Diphen, Diphenhist, Dytan, Siladryl, Sominex, Allerdryl, Nytol)*

▶LK ♀B ▶– $

ADULT – Allergic rhinitis, urticarial, hypersensitivity reactions: 25–50 mg PO/IM/IV q4–6h. Max 300–400 mg/day. Motion sickness: 25–50 mg PO pre-exposure and q4–6h prn.

Drug-induced parkinsonism: 10–50 mg IV/IM. Antitussive: 25 mg PO q4h. Max 100 mg/day EPS: 25–50 mg PO three to four times per day or 10–50 mg IV/IM three to four times per day. Insomnia: 25–50 mg PO at bedtime.

PEDS — Hypersensitivity reactions: Give 12.5–25 mg PO q4–6h or 5 mg/kg/day PO/IV/IM divided four times per day for age 6–11 yo, give adult dose for age 12 yo or older. Max 150 mg/day. Antitussive (syrup): Give 6.25 mg PO q4h (up to 25 mg/day) for age 2–5 yo, give 12.5 mg PO q4h (up to 50 mg/day) for age 6–12 yo. EPS: 12.5–25 mg PO three to four times per day or 5 mg/kg/day IV/IM divided four times per day, max 300 mg/day. Insomnia, age 12 yo or older: 25–50 mg PO at bedtime.

FORMS — OTC Trade only: Tabs 25, 50 mg. Chewable tabs 12.5 mg. OTC and RX: Generic only: Caps 25, 50 mg. Softgel cap 25 mg. OTC Generic/Trade: Soln 6.25 or 12.5 mg per 5 mL. Rx: Trade only: (Dytan) Susp 25 mg/mL. Chewable tabs 25 mg.

NOTES — Anticholinergic side effects are enhanced in the elderly and may worsen dementia or delirium. Avoid use with donepezil, rivastigmine, or galantamine.

MOA — Antihistamine.

ADVERSE EFFECTS — Serious: None. Frequent: Sedation, dry mouth.

[19]CHLORPROMAZINE

▶LK ♀?/?/? Animal data suggest possibility of embryotoxicity.
▶– $$$$$

ADULT — Psychotic Disorders: 10–25 mg PO two to four times per day or 25–50 mg IM, can repeat in 1 h. Severe acute psychosis may require 400 mg IM q4–6h up to max 2000 mg/day

IM. Intractable hiccups: 25–50 mg PO/IM three to four times per day. Persistent hiccups may require 25–50 mg in 0.5–1 liter NS by slow infusion.

PEDS – Severe behavioral problems/psychotic disorders, age 6 mo to 12 yo: 0.5 mg/kg PO q4–6h prn or 1 mg/kg PR q6–8h prn or 0.5 mg/kg IM q6–8h prn.

FORMS – Generic only: Tabs 10, 25, 50, 100, 200 mg.

NOTES – Monitor for hypotension with IM or IV use. Brand name Thorazine no longer available.

MOA – Low-potency dopamine antagonist.

ADVERSE EFFECTS – Serious: Seizures, neuroleptic malignant syndrome, extrapyramidal side effects, tardive dyskinesia, QT prolongation, jaundice. Frequent: Drowsiness, nausea, dry mouth, constipation, urinary retention, hypotension, headache, hyperprolactinemia.

[20] MAGNESIUM SULFATE

▶K ♀D C/D ▶+ $

ADULT – Hypomagnesemia: Mild deficiency: 1 g IM q6h for 4 doses; severe deficiency: 2 g IV over 1 h (monitor for hypotension). Hyperalimentation: Maintenance requirements not precisely known; adults generally require 8–24 mEq/day. Seizure prevention in severe preeclampsia or eclampsia: ACOG recommendations: 4–6 g IV loading dose then 1–2 g/h IV continuous infusion for at least 24 h. Or per product information: Total initial dose of 10–14 g administered via IV infusion and IM doses (4 g IV infusion with 5 g IM injections in each buttock). Initial dose is followed by 4–5 g IM into alternate buttocks q4h prn or initial dose is followed by 1–2 g/h constant IV infusion. Max: 30–40 g/24 h.

PEDS – Not approved in children.

UNAPPROVED ADULT – Preterm labor: 6 g IV over 20 min, then 1–3 g/h titrated to decrease contractions. Has been used as an adjunctive bronchodilator in very severe acute asthma (2 g IV over 10–20 min), and in chronic fatigue syndrome. Torsades de pointes: 1–2 g IV in D5W over 5–60 min.

UNAPPROVED PEDS – Hypomagnesemia: 25–50 mg/kg IV/IM q4–6h for 3–4 doses, max single dose 2 g. Hyperalimentation: Maintenance requirements not precisely known; infants require 2–10 mEq/day. Acute nephritis: 20–40 mg/kg (in 20% soln) IM prn. Adjunctive bronchodilator in very severe acute asthma: 25–100 mg/kg IV over 10–20 min.

NOTES – 1000 mg magnesium sulfate contains 8 mEq elem magnesium. Do not give faster than 1.5 mL/min (of 10% soln) except in eclampsia or seizures. Use caution in renal insufficiency, may accumulate. Monitor urine output, patellar reflex, respiratory rate, and serum magnesium level. Concomitant use with terbutaline may lead to fatal pulmonary edema. IM administration must be diluted to a 20% soln. If needed, may reverse toxicity with calcium gluconate 1 g IV. Continuous use in pregnancy beyond 5–7 days may cause fetal harm.

MOA – Essential mineral needed for muscle function, organ function, potassium and calcium absorption; blocks neuromuscular transmission to prevent or control convulsions.

ADVERSE EFFECTS – Serious: Magnesium intoxication (in recipient of drug or in newborn of pregnant woman receiving Mg), cardiac depression, respiratory paralysis, hypotension, stupor, hypothermia, circulatory collapse. Frequent: Flushing, sweating, depressed reflexes.

HEADACHE

²¹**VALPROIC ACID—NEUROLOGY** *(Depakene, Depakote, Depakote ER, Depacon, Stavzor, divalproex, sodium valproate, Epival, Deproic)*

▶L ♀D Category X when used for migraine prevention ▶+ $$$$

WARNING – Fatal hepatic failure reported, especially in children younger than 2 yo with comorbidities and on multiple anticonvulsants. Monitor LFTs during first 6 months of treatment and periodically thereafter. Should not be used in children under 2 yo. Life-threatening pancreatitis reported; evaluate for abdominal pain, N/V, and/or anorexia and discontinue if pancreatitis occurs. May be more teratogenic than other anticonvulsants (eg, carbamazepine, lamotrigine, and phenytoin) and is associated with neural tube defects, lower IQ in offspring, and other effects. Hepatic failure and clotting disorders have also occurred when used during pregnancy. Use during pregnancy when no other options, and provide effective contraception in women who may become pregnant.

ADULT – Epilepsy (complex partial seizures): 10–15 mg/kg/day PO or IV infusion over 60 min (rate no faster than 20 mg/min) in divided doses (immediate-release, delayed-release, or IV) or given once daily (Depakote ER). Increase by 5–10 mg/kg/day at weekly intervals to max 60 mg/kg/day. Simple and complex absence seizures: Start 15 mg/kg/day and increase weekly as needed by 5–10 mg/kg/day to max of 60 mg/kg/day. For both seizure types, give Depakote ER once daily. Give delayed-release products (Depakote, Depakote Sprinkles) in divided doses above 250 mg/day. Immediate-release products (Depakene, valproic acid) should be divided twice daily for

500 mg/day and above, and three times daily for doses of 750 mg and above. Migraine prophylaxis: Start 250 mg PO two times per day (Depakote or Stavzor) or 500 mg PO daily (Depakote ER) for 1 week, then increase to max 1000 mg/day PO divided two times per day (Depakote or Stavzor) or given once daily (Depakote ER).

PEDS — Epilepsy (complex partial seizures), ages 10 yo and older: 10–15 mg/kg/day PO or IV infusion over 60 min (rate no faster than 20 mg/min). Increase by 5–10 mg/kg/day at weekly intervals to max 60 mg/kg/day. Simple and complex absence seizures (ages 10 yo and older): Start 15 mg/kg/day and increase weekly as needed by 5–10 mg/kg/day to max dose 60 mg/kg/day. For both seizure types, give Depakote ER once daily. Give delayed-release products (Depakote, Depakote Sprinkles) in divided doses for doses above 250 mg/day. Immediate-release products (Depakene, valproic acid) should be divided twice daily for 500 mg/day and three times daily for doses of 750 mg and above.

UNAPPROVED ADULT — Status epilepticus (not first-line): Load 20–40 mg/kg IV (rate no faster than 6 mg/kg/min), then continue 4–8 mg/kg IV three times per day to achieve therapeutic level. May use lower loading dose if already on valproate.

UNAPPROVED PEDS — Status epilepticus, age older than 2 yo (not first-line): Load 20–40 mg/kg IV over 1–5 min, then 5 mg/kg/h adjusted to achieve therapeutic level. May use lower loading dose if already on valproate. Epilepsy (ages 2–under 10 yo): start 10–15 mg/kg/day PO or IV infusion over 60 min (rate no faster than 20 mg/min). Increase by 5–10 mg/kg/day at weekly intervals to max 60 mg/kg/day. IV administration should be divided every 6 h. Delayed-release products should be given in 2–3 daily doses. Immediate-release products (Depakene, valproic acid) should be divided twice daily for 500 mg/day and above, and three times daily for doses of 750 mg and above.

FORMS – Generic/Trade: Immediate-release caps 250 mg (Depakene), syrup (Depakene, valproic acid) 250 mg/5 mL. Delayed-release tabs (Depakote) 125, 250, 500 mg. Extended-release tabs (Depakote ER) 250, 500 mg. Delayed-release sprinkle caps (Depakote) 125 mg. Trade only (Stavzor): Delayed-release caps 125, 250, 500 mg.

NOTES – May be used for other seizure types in association with complex partial or absence seizures. Contraindicated in urea cycle disorders, hepatic dysfunction, in patients with genetic mutations in mitochondrial DNA polymerase gamma, and migraine prophylaxis in pregnant women. Usual therapeutic anticonvulsant trough level is 50–100 mcg/mL. Depakote and Depakote ER are not interchangeable. Depakote ER is approximately 10% less bioavailable than Depakote. Divalproex sodium is released over 8–12 h with Depakote (1–4 doses/day), and 18–24 h with Depakote ER (1 dose/day). Many drug interactions. Patients other anticonvulsants may require higher doses of valproic acid. Reduce dose in the elderly. Hyperammonemia (increased by concurrent topiramate), GI irritation, or thrombocytopenia may occur. Use lower initial dose, and titrate slower for patients on rufinamide. Carbapenem antibiotics may reduce serum concentration to ineffective levels.

MOA – May increase GABA levels and modulate sodium channels.

ADVERSE EFFECTS – Serious: Hepatotoxicity, anaphylaxis, polycystic ovarian syndrome, bone marrow suppression, thrombocytopenia, bleeding, pancreatitis, SIADH, Stevens-Johnson syndrome, DRESS, hyperammonemia, suicidality. Frequent: N/V, diarrhea, weight gain, CNS depression, drowsiness, tremor, alopecia, nystagmus, asthenia.

[22]DEXAMETHASONE *(DexPak, Dexamethasone Intensol, Dexasone)*

▶L ♀C ▶– $

ADULT – Anti-inflammatory/immunosuppressive: 0 5–9 g mg/day PO/IV/IM divided two to four times per day. Cerebral edema: 10–20 mg IV load, then 4 mg IM q6h (off-label IV use common) or 1–3 mg PO three times per day. Multiple sclerosis (acute exacerbation): 30 mg/day for 1 week, then 4–12 mg every other day for 1 mo.

PEDS – Dosing varies by indication; start 0.02–0.3 mg/kg/day divided three to four times per day.

UNAPPROVED ADULT – Initial treatment of immune thrombocytopenic purpura: 40 mg PO daily for 4 days. Fetal lung maturation, maternal antepartum between 24 and 34 weeks' gestation: 6 mg IM q12h for 4 doses. Bacterial meningitis (controversial): 0.15 mg/kg IV q6h for 2–4 days; start 10–15 min before first dose of antibiotic. Antiemetic, prophylaxis: 8 mg IV or 12 mg PO prior to chemotherapy; 8 mg PO daily for 2–4 days. Antiemetic, treatment: 10–20 mg PO/IV q4–6h.

UNAPPROVED PEDS – Anti-inflammatory/immunosuppressive: 0.08–0.3 mg/kg/day PO/IV/IM divided q6–12h. Croup: 0.6 mg/kg PO/IV/IM for one dose. Bacterial meningitis (controversial): 0.15 mg/kg IV q6h for 2–4 days; start 10–15 min before the first dose of antibiotic. Bronchopulmonary dysplasia in preterm infants: 0.5 mg/kg PO/IV divided q12h for 3 days, then taper. Acute asthma: Older than 2 yo: 0.6 mg/kg to max 16 mg PO daily for 2 days.

FORMS – Generic only: Tabs 0.5, 0.75, 1.0, 1.5, 2, 4, 6 mg; Elixir 0.5 mg/5 mL; Soln 0.5 mg/5 mL. Trade only: Tabs DexPak 13 day (51 total 1.5 mg tabs for a 13-day taper), DexPak 10 day (35 total 1.5 mg tabs for 10-day taper), DexPak 6 days (21 total 1.5 mg tabs for 6-day taper); Soln Dexamethasone Intensol 1 mg/1 mL (concentrate).

NOTES – Avoid prolonged use in children due to possible bone growth retardation. If such therapy necessary, monitor growth and development.

MOA – Long-acting glucocorticoid.

ADVERSE EFFECTS – Serious: Hypertension, diabetes, osteoporosis, immunosuppression, impaired wound healing, adrenal suppression, peptic ulcer disease, cataracts. Frequent: Cushingoid state, N/V, weight gain, myopathy, leukocytosis, skin atrophy, edema.

[23]HALOPERIDOL *(Haldol)*

▶LK ♀??? There is evidence in humans for limb malformations when used in the first trimester. Exposure in 3rd trimester associated with withdrawal/extrpyramidal effects. ▶– $$$ ■

ADULT – Psychotic disorders and Tourette syndrome: 0.5–5 mg PO two to three times per day. Usual effective dose is 6–20 mg/day, max dose is 100 mg/day PO or 2–5 mg IM every 1–8 h prn to max 20 mg/day IM. May use long-acting (depot) formulation when patients are stabilized on a fixed daily dose. Approximate conversion ratio: 100–200 mg IM (depot) q4 weeks is equivalent to 10 mg/day PO haloperidol.

PEDS — Psychotic disorders, age 3–12 yo: 0.05 mg to 0.15 mg/kg/day PO divided two to three times per day. Tourette syndrome or nonpsychotic disorders, age 3–12 yo: 0.05 mg to 0.075 mg/kg/day PO divided two to three times per day. Increase dose by 0.5 mg every week to max dose of 6 mg/day. Not approved for IM administration in children.

UNAPPROVED ADULT — Acute psychosis and combative behavior: 5–10 mg IV/IM, repeat prn in 10–30 min. IV route associated with QT prolongation, torsades de pointes, and sudden death; use ECG monitoring.

UNAPPROVED PEDS — Psychosis, age 6–12 yo: 1–3 mg/dose IM (as lactate) q4–8h, max 0.15 mg/kg/day.

FORMS — Generic only: Tabs 0.5, 1, 2, 5, 10, 20 mg.

NOTES — Therapeutic range is 2–15 ng/mL.

MOA — High-potency dopamine antagonist.

ADVERSE EFFECTS — Serious: Seizures, neuroleptic malignant syndrome, extrapyramidal side effects, tardive dyskinesia, QT prolongation, sudden death, jaundice, rhabdomyolysis. Frequent: Drowsiness, nausea, dry mouth, constipation, urinary retention, hypotension, headache, hyperprolactinemia.

[24]PROPOFOL *(Diprivan)*

▶L ♀B ▶– $

WARNING — Beware of respiratory depression/apnea. Administer with appropriate monitoring.

ADULT — Anesthesia (age younger than 55 yo): 40 mg IV q10 sec until induction onset (typical 2–2.5 mg/kg). Follow with maintenance infusion generally 100–200 mcg/kg/min. Lower doses in elderly or for sedation. ICU ventilator sedation: Infusion 5–50 mcg/kg/min.

PEDS — Anesthesia age 3 yo or older: 2.5–3.5 mg/kg IV over 20–30 sec, followed with infusion 125–300 mcg/kg/min. Not recommended if age younger than 3 yo or for prolonged ICU use.

UNAPPROVED ADULT — Deep sedation: 1 mg/kg IV over 20–30 sec. Repeat 0.5 mg/kg IV prn. Intubation adjunct: 2.0–2.5 mg/kg IV.

UNAPPROVED PEDS — Deep sedation: 1 mg/kg IV (max 40 mg) over 20–30 sec. Repeat 0.5 mg/kg (max 20 mg) IV prn.

NOTES — Avoid with egg or soy allergies. Prolonged infusions may lead to hypertriglyceridemia. Injection pain can be treated or pretreated with lidocaine 40–50 mg IV.

MOA — Nonbarbiturate hypnotic without analgesic properties.

ADVERSE EFFECTS — Serious: Respiratory depression, hypotension, hypersensitivity. Frequent: Injection site pain, sedation.

[25]KETAMINE *(Ketalar)*

▶L ♀C ▷? ©III $■

WARNING — Post-anesthetic emergence reactions up to 24 h later manifested as dreamlike state, vivid imagery, hallucinations, and delirium reported in about 12% of cases. Incidence reduced when (1) age less than 15 yo or greater than 65 yo, (2) concomitant use of benzodiazepines, lower dose, or used as induction agent only (because of use of post-intubation sedation).

ADULT — Induction of anesthesia: Adult: 1–2 mg/kg IV over 1–2 min (produces 5–10 min dissociative state) or 6.5–13 mg/kg IM (produces 10–20 min dissociative state).

PEDS — Age over 16 yo: same as adult.

UNAPPROVED ADULT — Dissociative sedation: 1–2 mg/kg IV over 1–2 min (sedation lasting 10–20 min); repeat 0.5 mg/kg doses q5–15 min may be given; 4–5 mg/kg IM (sedation lasting 15–30 min); repeat 2–4 mg/kg IM can be given if needed after 10–15 min. Analgesia adjunct subdissociative dose: 0.01–0.5 mg/kg in conjunction with opioid analgesia.

UNAPPROVED PEDS – Dissociative sedation: Age older than 3 mo: 1–2 mg/kg IV (produces 5–10 min dissociative state) over 1–2 min or 4–5 mg/kg IM (produces 10–20 min dissociative state). Not approved for age younger than 3 mo.

FORMS – Generic/Trade: 10, 50, 100 mg/mL.

NOTES – Recent evidence suggests ketamine is not contraindicated in patients with head injuries. However, avoid if CAD or severe HTN. Concurrent administration of atropine no longer recommended. Consider prophylactic ondansetron to reduce vomiting and prophylactic midazolam (0.3 mg/kg) to reduce recovery reactions.

MOA – NMDA receptor antagonist that produces dissociative state.

ADVERSE EFFECTS – Serious: Laryngospasm, hallucinatory emergence reactions, hypersalivation. Frequent: Nystagmus, hypertension, tachycardia, N/V, muscular hypertonicity, myoclonus.

---

[26]ACETYLSALICYLIC ACID (Ecotrin, Empirin, Halfprin, Bayer, Anacin, ZORprin, Aspirin, Asaphen, Entrophen, Novasen)

▶K ❸ ♀D ▶? $

ADULT – Mild to moderate pain, fever: 325–650 mg PO/PR q4h pm. Acute rheumatic fever: 5–8 g/day, initially. RA/OA: 3.2–6 g/day in divided doses. Platelet aggregation inhibition: 81–325 mg PO daily.

PEDS – Mild to moderate pain, fever: 10–15 mg/kg/dose PO q4–6h not to exceed 60–80 mg/kg/day. JRA: 60–100 mg/kg/day PO divided q6–8h. Acute rheumatic fever: 100 mg/kg/day PO/PR for 2 weeks, then 75 mg/kg/day for 4–6 weeks. Kawasaki disease: 80–100 mg/kg/day divided four times per day PO/PR until fever resolves, then 3–5 mg/kg/day PO q AM for 7 weeks or longer if there is ECG evidence of coronary artery abnormalities.

UNAPPROVED ADULT – Primary prevention of cardiovascular events: 10-year CHD risk more than 6–10% based on Framingham risk scoring): 75–325 mg PO daily. Post ST-elevation MI: 162–325 mg PO on day 1, continue indefinitely at 75–162 mg/day. Post non-ST elevation MI: 162–325 mg PO on day 1, continue indefinitely at 75–162 mg/day. Long-term antithrombotic therapy for chronic A-fib/flutter in patients with low to moderate risk of CVA (age younger than 75 yo without risk factors): 325 mg PO daily. Percutaneous coronary intervention pretreatment: Already taking daily aspirin therapy: 75–325 mg PO before procedure. Not already taking daily aspirin therapy: 300–325 mg PO at least 2–24 h before procedure. Post-percutaneous coronary intervention: 325 mg daily in combination with clopidogrel for at least 1 month after bare metal stent placement, at least 3–6 months after drug-eluting stent placement; then 75–162 mg PO daily indefinitely. Post-percutaneous coronary brachytherapy: 75–325 mg daily in combination with clopidogrel indefinitely.

FORMS – Generic/Trade (OTC): Tabs 325, 500 mg; chewable 81 mg; enteric-coated 81, 162 mg (Halfprin), 81, 325, 500 mg

(Ecotrin), 65G; 975 mg. Trade only; Tabs, controlled-release 650, 800 mg (ZORprin, Rx). Generic only (OTC): Supps 60, 120, 200, 300, 600 mg.

NOTES — Consider discontinuation 1 week prior to surgery (except coronary bypass or in first year post-coronary stent implantation) because of the possibility of postop bleeding. Aspirin intolerance occurs in 4% to 19% of asthmatics. Use caution in liver damage, renal insufficiency, peptic ulcer, or bleeding tendencies. Crush or chew tabs (including enteric-coated products) in first dose with acute MI. Higher doses of aspirin (1.3 g/day) have not been shown to be superior to low doses in preventing TIAs and CVAs.

MOA — Anti-inflammatory, antipyretic, analgesic. Inhibits prostaglandin synthesis and platelet aggregation by inactivating the enzyme cyclooxygenase.

ADVERSE EFFECTS — Serious: Hypersensitivity, Reye's syndrome, GI bleeding, nephrotoxicity. Frequent: Nausea, dyspepsia, tinnitus (large doses), dizziness (large doses).

[27]RIZATRIPTAN *(Maxalt, Maxalt MLT)*

▶LK ♀C ▶? $$$

ADULT — Migraine treatment: 5–10 mg PO; may repeat 2 h prn: Max 30 mg/24 h.

PEDS — Migraine treatment: Children 6–17 yo, 5 mg PO if < 40 kg and 10 mg PO for 40 kg and above. Do not give more than one dose in 24 h.

FORMS — Generic/Trade: Tabs 5, 10 mg. Orally disintegrating tabs 5, 10 mg.

NOTES — Should not be combined with MAOIs. MLT form dissolves on tongue without liquids. Adult patients receiving propranolol should only receive 5 mg dose and not more than 3 doses per 24 h. For pediatric patients taking propranolol and weighing more than 40 kg only a 5 mg dose one time in 24 h should be used. Do not give to children weighing less than 40 kg and taking propranolol.

MOA – Serotonin 5–HT1B/D agonist.

ADVERSE EFFECTS – Serious: Chest pain/tightness, coronary vasospasm, acute MI, arrhythmias, peripheral ischemia, stroke, HTN, medication overuse headache, serotonin syndrome. Frequent: Asthenia, fatigue, drowsiness, pain/pressure sensation, dizziness, paresthesia.

MUSCULOSKELETAL PAIN (TRAUMATIC/NON-TRAUMATIC)

Inpatient Analgesics (in the ED)	Outpatient Analgesics (discharge)
Non-Opioid	**Non-Opioid**
Oral Regimen: [1]**Acetaminophen:** 500 mg, best if combined with [2]**Ibuprofen:** 400 mg, or [3]**Naproxen:** 500 mg, or [4]**Diclofenac:** 50 mg, or [5]**Ketorolac:** 10 mg The following three medications should be used only with proven muscle spasm. They are not to be administered for routine treatment of musculoskeletal pain: [6]**PO Methocarbamol:** 500–1500 mg [7]**Cyclobenzaprine:** 5–10 mg [8]**PO Orphenadrine:** 100 mg	[2]**PO Ibuprofen:** 400 mg q8h × 3 days (max 5 days with 1200 mg/d). [3]**PO Naproxen:** 500 mg q12h × 3 days (max 5 days). [4]**PO Diclofenac:** 50 mg q8h × 3 days (max 5 days). [1]**PO Acetaminophen:** 500 mg PO q8h × 3 days (max 1500 mg/day). Best if combined with [2]**Ibuprofen** at 400 mg q8h or [3]**Naproxen** at 500 mg q12h. [18]**PO Diflunisal** (Dolobid): 250–500 mg PO q12h × 3 days.

(*continues*)

Inpatient Analgesics (in the ED)	Outpatient Analgesics (discharge)
Non-Opioid	**Non-Opioid**

<u>Topical Regimen:</u> [9]**Topical Diclofenac Patch (Gel):** a single patch or thin layer to the affected area. [10]**Topical Lidocaine** (4–5% patch, 2% cream): up to two patches or thin layer of cream to the affected area. [11]**Topical Capsaicin** (0.025–0.15% cream): apply thin layer to affected area. <u>Trigger Point Injection:</u> up to 10 mL of 0.5% [12]**Bupivacaine**, or 10 mL of 1% [13]**Lidocaine** to site of maximal pain. <u>Regional Anesthesia (UGRA):</u> [12]**Bupivacaine** w/o epi: 0.25–0.5%, max 2.5 mg/kg. [12]**Bupivacaine** with epi: 0.25–0.5%, max 3.0 mg/kg. [13]**Lidocaine** w/o epi: 0.5–2%, 4.5 mg/kg, max 300 mg. [13]**Lidocaine** with epi: 0.5–2%, 7 mg/kg, max 500 mg. [14]**Chloroprocaine** 2–3%, max 11 mg/kg.	**The following three medications should only be used with proven muscle spasm. They are not to be administered for routine treatment of musculoskeletal pain:** [6]**PO Methocarbamol:** 500 mg q6–8h for 2–3 days, or [7]**Cyclobenzaprine:** 5–10 mg (start with 5 mg in elderly) × 2–3 days, or [8]**PO Orphenadrine:** 100 mg PO two times per day × 2–3 days. <u>Topical Regimen:</u> [9]**Topical Diclofenac Gel/ Patch:** Apply patch to affected area q12h for 5–7 days. [10]**Topical Lidocaine** (4–5% patch, 2% cream): apply up to 2 patches to affected area for 12 h, then 12-h patch-free period.

(*continues*)

Inpatient Analgesics (in the ED)	Outpatient Analgesics (discharge)
Non-Opioid	**Non-Opioid**
[15]**Ropivacaine:** 0.2–1%, max 3 mg/kg. **Parenteral Regimen:** [5]**IV Ketorolac:** 10–15 mg IVP (analgesic ceiling dose). [13]**IV Lidocaine:** 1.5 mg/kg of 2% (preservative-free lidocaine-cardiac or pre-made bags only) over 15 minutes (max dose 200 mg). [1]**IV Acetaminophen:** 1 g over 15 min (as adjunct to opioid/non-opioid) if patients are NPO/NPR or contraindications to opioids, NSAIDs, lidocaine or ketamine. [16]**Ketamine (Subdissociative Dose, SDK)** • **IV:** 0.3 mg/kg over 15 min, +/– continuous IV infusion at 0.15–0.2 mg/kg/h • **SQ** 0.3 mg/kg over 15 min, +/– continuous SQ infusion at 0.15–0.2 mg/kg/h	[11]**Topical Capsaicin** (0.025–0.15% cream): apply q12h to affected area × 5–7 days. Avoid contact with mucous membranes.

(continues)

Inpatient Analgesics (in the ED)	Outpatient Analgesics (discharge)
Non-Opioid	**Non-Opioid**
• **Intranasal (IN):** 0.5–1 mg/ kg (weight-based) q5–10 min (consider using highly concentrated solutions: Adults: 100 mg/mL Peds: 50 mg/mL; No more than 0.3–0.5 mL/per nostril). • **Inhalation:** [17]**Nitrous Oxide:** 50/50 mix, max 70/30 mix (single agent for mild painful procedures, adjunct to opioids, non-opioids, regional/ hematoma blocks).	
Opioid	**Opioid**
Opioids should not be routinely used in the ED for acute musculoskeletal pain. Every effort should be made to utilize non-pharmacological and non-opioid analgesics first and resort to opioids when pain is intractable and/or multidrug resistant, is related to severe traumatic injuries (fractures, dislocations), non-opioid analgesia failed to achieve an acceptable pain relief, and	Opioids should not be routinely used in the ED for acute musculoskeletal pain. Every effort should be made to utilize non-pharmacological and non-opioid analgesics first and resort to opioids when pain is intractable and/or multidrug resistant, is related to severe traumatic injuries (fractures, dislocations),

(continues)

Inpatient Analgesics (in the ED)	Outpatient Analgesics (discharge)
Opioid	**Opioid**
when benefits of their use outweigh the risks. When these agents are considered, frequent titration must be used. **Oral Regimen:** [19]**Morphine:** PO, Morphine Sulfate Immediate Release (MSIR): 15 mg. [20]**Fentanyl:** Transbuccal 100–200 µg dissolvable tablets, repeat at 60 min if pain persists. [21]**Hydromorphone** 2 mg. **Parenteral Regimen:** [19]**Morphine:** • **IV:** 0.05–0.1 mg/kg (weight-based), titrate q10–20 min. • **IV:** 4–6 mg (fixed), titrate q10–20 min. • **SQ:** 4–6 mg (fixed), re-administer as needed q30–40 min. • **IM:** 4–6 mg (fixed), re-administer as needed at q30–40 min (IM route should be avoided due to pain upon injection, muscle fibrosis, necrosis, increase in dosing requirements).	non-opioid analgesia failed to achieve an acceptable pain relief, and when benefits of their use outweigh the risks. When these agents are considered, lowest effective dose and shortest course must be used. [19]**Morphine Sulfate Immediate Release (MSIR):** 15 mg q6–8h × 2–3 days (opioid-naïve patients). [23]**Hydrocodone/ Acetaminophen (Norco):** 5/325 mg: 1–2 tabs q6–8h × 2–3 days. [24]**Hydrocodone/ Acetaminophen (Vicodin, Lortab, Lorcet):** 5/300 mg: 1–2 tabs q6–8h × 2–3 days. [25]**Hydrocodone/Ibuprofen (Vicoprofen):** 5/200 mg: 1–2 tabs q6–8h × 2–3 days.

MUSCULOSKELETAL PAIN (Traumatic/Non-Traumatic)

(continues)

Inpatient Analgesics (in the ED)	Outpatient Analgesics (discharge)
Opioid	**Opioid**
Nebulized (via Breath Actuated Nebulizer [BAN]): Adults: 10–20 mg (fixed), repeat q15–20 min up to three doses Peds: 0.2–0.4 mg/kg (weight-based), repeat q15–20 min up to three doses • **PCA:** Demand dose: 1–2 mg Continuous basal infusion: 0.5–2 mg/h [20]**Fentanyl:** • **IV:** 0.25–0.5 µg/kg (weight-based), titrate q10 min. • **IV:** 25–50 µg (fixed), titrate q10 min. **Nebulized** (via BAN): • Adults: 2–4 µg/kg (weight-based), titrate q20–30 min, up to three doses Peds: 2–4 µg/kg (weight-based), titrate q20–30 min, up to three doses	[26]**Oxycodone/ Acetaminophen (Percocet, Roxicet):** 5/325 mg: 1–2 tabs q6–8h × 2–3 days. [21]**Hydromorphone:** 2–4 mg q6–8h × 2–3 days (for opioid-naïve patients start with 2 mg dose).

(continues)

Inpatient Analgesics (in the ED)	Outpatient Analgesics (discharge)
Opioid	Opioid
• **Intranasal (IN):** 1–2 μg/kg (weight-based), titrate q5–10 min (consider using highly concentrated solutions: Adults: 100 μg/mL, Peds: 50 μg/mL. No more than 0.3–0.5 mL/per nostril). • **Transmucosal:** 10–20 mcg/kg lollipops • **PCA:** Demand dose: 20–50 μg Continuous basal infusion: 0.05–0.1 μg/kg/h. [21]**Hydromorphone:** • **IV:** 0.2–0.5 mg initial, titrate q10–15 min. • **SQ:** 0.5–1 mg, titrate q30–40 min. • **IM:** 0.5–1 mg, titrate q30–40 min (IM route should be avoided due to pain, muscle fibrosis, necrosis, increase in dosing requirements).	

(continues)

Inpatient Analgesics (in the ED)	Outpatient Analgesics (discharge)
Opioid	Opioid
• **PCA:** Demand dose: 0.2–0.4 mg Continuous basal infusion: 0.1–0.4 mg/h [22]**Sufentanil:** • **Intranasal (IN):** 0.5 µg/kg, titration q10 min up to three doses	

[1]**ACETAMINOPHEN** *(Tylenol, Panadol, Tempra, Ofirmev, Paracetamol, Abenol, Atasol, Pediatrix)*

▶LK ♀B ▶+ $

ADULT – Analgesic/antipyretic: 325–1000 mg PO q4–6h prn. 650 mg PR q4–6h pm. Max dose 4 g/day. OA: Extended-release: 2 caps PO q8h around the clock. Max dose 6 caps/day.
PEDS – Analgesic/antipyretic: 10–15 mg/kg q4–6h PO/PR pm. Max 5 doses/day.
UNAPPROVED ADULT – OA: 1000 mg PO four times per day.
FORMS – OTC: Tabs 325, 500, 650 mg. Chewable tabs 80 mg. Orally disintegrating tabs 80, 160 mg. Caps/gelcaps 500 mg. Extended-release caplets 650 mg. Liquid 160 mg/5 mL, 500 mg/15 mL. Supps 80, 120, 325, 650 mg.

[2]IBUPROFEN *(Motrin, Advil, Nuprin, Rufen, NeoProfen, Caldolor)*

▶L ⊗ ♀B (D in 3rd trimester) ▶+ ■

ADULT — RA/OA, gout: 200–800 mg PO three to four times per day. Mild to moderate pain: 400 mg PO q4–6h. 400–800 mg IV (Caldolor) q6h prn. 400 mg IV (Caldolor) q4–6h or 100–200 mg q4h prn. Primary dysmenorrhea: 400 mg PO q4h prn. Fever: 200 mg PO q4–6h prn. Migraine pain: 200–400 mg PO not to exceed 400 mg in 24 h unless directed by a physician (OTC dosing). Max dose 3.2 g/day.

PEDS — JRA: 30–50 mg/kg/day PO divided q6h. Max dose 2400 mg/24 h. 20 mg/kg/day may be adequate for milder disease. Analgesic/antipyretic, age older than 6 mo: 5–10 mg/kg PO q6–8h, prn. Max dose 40 mg/kg/day. Patent ductus arteriosus in neonates 32 weeks' gestational age or younger weighing 500–1500 g (NeoProfen): Specialized dosing.

FORMS — OTC: Caps/Liqui-Gel caps 200 mg. Tabs 100, 200 mg. Chewable tabs 100 mg. Susp (infant gtts) 50 mg/1.25 mL (with calibrated dropper), 100 mg/5 mL. Rx Generic/Trade: Tabs 400, 600, 800 mg.

NOTES — May antagonize antiplatelet effects of aspirin if given simultaneously. Take aspirin 2 h prior to ibuprofen. Administer IV (Caldolor) over at least 30 min; hydration important.

MOA — Anti-inflammatory/antipyretic, analgesic.

ADVERSE EFFECTS — Serious: Hypersensitivity, GI bleeding, nephrotoxicity. Frequent: Nausea, dyspepsia.

[3]NAPROXEN *(Naprosyn, Aleve, Anaprox, EC-Naprosyn, Naprelan, Prevacid, NapraPAC)*

▶L ⊗ ♀B (D in 3rd trimester) ▶+ $■

WARNING – Multiple strengths; see FORMS and write specific product on Rx.

ADULT – RA/OA, ankylosing spondylitis, pain, dysmenorrhea, acute tendinitis and bursitis, fever: 250–500 mg PO two times per day. Delayed-release: 375–500 mg PO two times per day (do not crush or chew). Controlled-release: 750–1000 mg PO daily. Acute gout: 750 mg PO once, then 250 mg PO q8h until the attack subsides. Controlled-release: 1000–1500 mg PO once, then 1000 mg PO daily until the attack subsides.

PEDS – JRA: 10–20 mg/kg/day PO divided two times per day (up to 1250 mg/24 h). Pain for age older than 2 yo: 5–7 mg/kg/dose PO q8–12h.

UNAPPROVED ADULT – Acute migraine: 750 mg PO once, then 250–500 mg PO pm. Migraine prophylaxis, menstrual migraine: 500 mg PO two times per day beginning 1 day prior to onset of menses and ending on last day of period.

FORMS – OTC Generic/Trade (Aleve): Tabs, immediate-release 200 mg. OTC Trade only (Aleve): Caps, Gelcaps, immediate-release 200 mg. Rx Generic/Trade: Tabs, immediate-release (Naprosyn) 250, 375, 500 mg. (Anaprox) 275, 550 mg. Tabs, delayed-release enteric-coated (EC-Naprosyn) 375, 500 mg. Tabs, controlled-release (Naprelan) 375, 500, 750 mg. Susp (Naprosyn) 125 mg/5 mL. Prevacid NapraPAC: 7 lansoprazole 15 mg caps packaged with 14 naproxen tabs 375 mg or 500 mg.

NOTES – All dosing is based on naproxen content: 500 mg naproxen is equivalent to 550 mg naproxen sodium.

MOA – Anti-inflammatory, analgesic.
ADVERSE EFFECTS – Serious: Hypersensitivity, GI bleeding, nephrotoxicity. Frequent: Nausea, dyspepsia.

[4]DICLOFENAC *(Voltaren, Voltaren XR, Flector, Zipsor, Cambia, Zorvolex, Voltaren Rapide)*

▶L ⊘ ♀B (D in 3rd trimester) ▶– $$$■

WARNING – Multiple strengths; see FORMS and write specific product on Rx.

ADULT – OA: Immediate- or delayed-release: 50 mg PO two to three times per day or 75 mg two times per day. Extended-release 100 mg PO daily. Gel: Apply 4 g to knees or 2 g to hands four times per day using enclosed dosing card. RA: Immediate- or delayed-release 50 mg PO three to four times per day or 75 mg two times per day. Extended-release 100 mg PO one to two times per day. Ankylosing spondylitis: Immediate- or delayed-release 25 mg PO four times per day and at bedtime. Analgesia and primary dysmenorrhea: Immediate- or delayed-release 50 mg PO three times per day. Acute pain in of strains, sprains, or contusions: Apply 1 patch to painful area two times per day. Acute migraine with or without aura: 50 mg single dose (Cambia), mix packet with 30–60 mL water.
PEDS – Not approved in children.

UNAPPROVED PEDS – JRA: 2–3 mg/kg/day PO.

FORMS – Generic/Trade: Tabs, extended-release (Voltaren XR) 100 mg. Topical gel (Voltaren) 1% 100 g tube. Generic only: Tabs, immediate-release: 25, 50 mg. Generic only: Tabs, delayed-release: 25, 50, 75 mg. Trade only: Patch (Flector) 1.3% diclofenac epolamine. Trade only: Caps, liquid-filled (Zipsor)

25 mg. Caps (Zorvolex) 18, 35 mg. Trade only: Powder for oral soln (Cambia) 50 mg.

NOTES — Check LFTs at baseline, within 4–8 weeks of initiation, then periodically. Do not apply patch to damaged or nonintact skin. Wash hands and avoid eye contact when handling the patch. Do not wear patch while bathing or showering.

MOA — Anti-inflammatory, analgesic.

ADVERSE EFFECTS — Serious: Hypersensitivity, GI bleeding, hepato/nephrotoxicity. Frequent: Nausea, dyspepsia, pruritus, and dermatitis with patch and gel.

[5]KETOROLAC *(Toradol)*

▶L ⊗♀B (D in 3rd trimester) ▶+ $$■

WARNING — Indicated for short-term (up to 5 days) therapy only. Ketorolac is a potent NSAID and can cause serious GI and renal adverse effects. It may also increase the risk of bleeding by inhibiting platelet function. Contraindicated in patients with active peptic ulcer disease, recent GI bleeding or perforation, a history of peptic ulcer disease or GI bleeding, or advanced renal impairment.

ADULT — Moderately severe, acute pain, single-dose treatment: 30–60 mg IM or 15–30 mg IV. Multiple-dose treatment: 15–30 mg IV/IM q6h IV/IM doses are not to exceed 60 mg/day for age 65 yo or older, wt < 50 kg, and patients with moderately elevated serum creatinine. Oral continuation therapy: 1.0 mg PO q4–6h prn, max dose 40 mg/day. Combined duration IV/IM and PO is not to exceed 5 days.

PEDS — Not approved in children.

UNAPPROVED PEDS — Pain: 0.5 mg/kg/dose IM/IV q6h (up to 30 mg q6h or 120 mg/day), give 10 mg PO qGh pm (up to 40 mg/day) for wt > 50 kg.

FORMS – Generic only: Tabs 10 mg.
MOA – Serious: Hypersensitivity, GI bleeding, nephrotoxicity. Frequent: Nausea, dyspepsia.

[6]METHOCARBAMOL *(Robaxin, Robaxin-750)*

▶LK ♀C ▶? $

ADULT – Musculoskeletal pain, acute relief: 1500 mg PO four times per day or 1000 mg IM/IV three times per day for 48–72h. Maintenance: 1000 mg PO four times per day, 750 mg PO q4h, or 1500 mg PO three times per day. Tetanus: Specialized dosing.
PEDS – Tetanus: Specialized dosing.
FORMS – Generic/Trade: Tabs 500, 750 mg. OTC in Canada.
NOTES – Max IV rate of undiluted drug 3 mL/min to avoid syncope, hypotension, and bradycardia. Total parenteral dosage should not exceed 3 g/day for more than 3 consecutive days, except in the treatment of tetanus. Urine may turn brown, black, or green.
MOA – Skeletal muscle relaxant.
ADVERSE EFFECTS – Serious: Syncope, hypotension. Frequent: Drowsiness, dizziness, discolored urine (brown, black, green).

[7]CYCLOBENZAPRINE *(Amrix, Flexeril, Fexmid)*

▶LK ♀B ▶? $

ADULT – Musculoskeletal pain: 5–10 mg PO three times per day up to max dose of 30 mg/day or 15–30 mg (extended-release) PO daily. Not recommended in elderly or for use longer than 2–3 weeks.
PEDS – Not approved in children.
FORMS – Generic/Trade: Tabs 5, 7.5, 10 mg. Extended-release caps 15, 30 mg ($$$$$).

NOTES – Contraindicated with recent or concomitant MAOI use, immediately post-MI, in patients with arrhythmias, conduction disturbances, heart failure, and hyperthyroidism. Not effective for cerebral or spinal cord disease or in children with cerebral palsy. May have similar adverse effects and drug interactions to TCAs. Caution with urinary retention, angle-closure glaucoma, increased intraocular pressure.

MOA – Skeletal muscle relaxant.

ADVERSE EFFECTS – Serious: Arrhythmia. Frequent: Drowsiness, dizziness, dry mouth, blurred vision.

[8]ORPHENADRINE *(Norflex)*

▶LK ♀C ▶? $$

ADULT – Musculoskeletal pain: 100 mg PO two times per day. 60 mg IV/IM two times per day.

PEDS – Not approved in children.

UNAPPROVED ADULT – Leg cramps: 100 mg PO at bedtime.

FORMS – Generic only: 100 mg extended-release. OTC in Canada.

NOTES – Contraindicated in glaucoma, pyloric or duodenal obstruction, BPH, and myasthenia gravis. Some products contain sulfites, which may cause allergic reactions. May increase anticholinergic effects of amantadine and decrease therapeutic effects of phenothiazines. Side effects include dry mouth, urinary retention and hesitancy, constipation, headache, and GI upset.

MOA – Skeletal muscle relaxant.

ADVERSE EFFECTS – Serious: Hypersensitivity, syncope. Frequent: Dry mouth, dizziness, constipation.

[9]DICLOFENAC-TOPICAL *(Solaraze, Voltaren, Pennsaid)*

▶L ♀C Category D at 30 weeks, gestation and beyond. Avoid use starting at 30 weeks' gestation. ▶? $$$

WARNING — Risk of cardiovascular and GI events.

ADULT — Osteoarthritis of areas amenable to topical therapy: 2 g (upper extremities) to 4 g (lower extremities) four times per day (Voltaren). 40 gtts to knee(s) four times daily.

PEDS — Not approved in children.

FORMS — Generic/Trade: Gel 3% (Solaraze) 100 g. Soln 1.5% (Pennsaid) 150 mL. Trade only: Gel 1% (Voltaren) 100 g. Soln 2.0% Pump (Pennsaid) 112 g.

NOTES — Avoid exposure to sun and sunlamps. Use caution in aspirin-sensitive patients. When using for OA (Voltaren), max daily dose 16 g to any single lower extremity joint, 8 g to any single upper extremity joint. Avoid use in setting of aspirin allergy or CABG surgery.

MOA — Inhibits prostaglandins at level of cyclooxygenase.

ADVERSE EFFECTS — Frequent: Rash, abdominal cramps, nausea, indigestion.

[10]LIDOCAINE—TOPICAL *(Xylocaine, Lidoderm, Numby Stuff, LMX, Zingo, Maxilene)*

▶LK ♀B ▶+ $

WARNING — Contraindicated in allergy to amide-type anesthetics.

ADULT — Topical anesthesia: Apply to affected area prn. Dose varies with anesthetic procedure, degree of anesthesia required, and individual patient response. Post-herpetic neuralgia (patch): Apply up to 3 patches to affected area at once for up to 12 h within a 24 h period.

PEDS – Topical anesthesia: Apply to affected area prn. Dose varies with anesthetic procedure, degree of anesthesia required, and individual patient response. Max 3 mg/kg/dose, do not repeat dose within 2 h. Intradermal powder injection for venipuncture/IV cannulation, for age 3–18 yo (Zingo): 0.5 mg to site 1–10 min prior.

UNAPPROVED PEDS – Topical anesthesia prior to venipuncture: Apply 30 min prior to procedure (ELA-Max 4%).

FORMS – For membranes of mouth and pharynx: Spray 10%, oint 5%, liquid 5%, soln 2%, 4% dental patch. For urethral use: Jelly 2%. Patch (Lidoderm $$$$$) 5%. Intradermal powder injection system: 0.5 mg (Zingo). OTC Trade only: Liposomal lidocaine 4% (ELA-Max).

NOTES – Apply patches only to intact skin to cover the most painful area. Patches may be cut into smaller sizes with scissors prior to removal of the release liner. Store and dispose out of the reach of children and pets to avoid possible toxicity from ingestion.

MOA – Anesthetic.

ADVERSE EFFECTS – Frequent: Skin irritation. Severe: CNS effects, bradycardia, bronchospasm, hypotension, allergic reactions.

[11]CAPSAICIN *(Zostrix, Zostrix-HP, Qutenza)*

▶? ♀? ▶? $

ADULT – Pain due to RA, OA, and neuralgias such as zoster or diabetic neuropathies: Apply to affected area up to three to four times per day. Post-herpetic neuralgia: 1 patch (Qutenza) applied for 1 h in medical office, may repeat every 3 months.

PEDS – Children older than 2 yo: Pain due to RA, OA, and neuralgias such as zoster or diabetic neuropathies: Apply to affected area up to three to four times per day.

UNAPPROVED ADULT – Psoriasis and intractable pruritus, post-mastectomy/post-amputation neuromas (phantom limb pain), vulvar vestibulitis, apocrine chromhidrosis, and reflex sympathetic dystrophy.

FORMS – Rx: Patch 8% (Qutenza). OTC: Generic/Trade: Cream 0.025% 60 g, 0.075% (HP) 60 g. OTC Generic only: Lotion 0.025% 59 mL, 0.075% 59 mL.

NOTES – Burning occurs in 30% or more of patients but diminishes with continued use. Pain more commonly occurs when applied less than three to four times per day. Wash hands immediately after application.

MOA – Counter-irritant, releases substance P.

ADVERSE EFFECTS – Frequent: Burning, redness, sensation of warmth.

[12]BUPIVACAINE (Marcaine, Sensorcaine)

▶LK ♀C ▷? $■

ADULT – Local anesthesia, nerve block: 0.25% injection. Up to 2.5 mg/kg without epinephrine and up 3.0 mg/kg with epinephrine.

PEDS – Not recommended in children younger than 12 yo.

FORMS – 0.25%, 0.5%, 0.75%, all with or without epinephrine.

NOTES – Onset 5 min, duration 2–4 h (longer with epi). Amide group.

MOA – Amide local anesthetic.

ADVERSE EFFECTS – Serious: Seizures, cardiovascular depression, bradycardia, hypersensitivity, methemoglobinemia. Frequent: None.

[13] LIDOCAINE—LOCAL ANESTHETIC (*Xylocaine*)

▶LK ♀B ▶? $

ADULT – Without epinephrine: Max dose 4.5 mg/kg not to exceed 300 mg. With epinephrine: Max dose 7 mg/kg not to exceed 500 mg. Dose for regional block varies by region.

PEDS – Same as adult.

FORMS – 0.5, 1, 1.5, 2%. With epi: 0.5, 1, 1.5, 2%.

NOTES – Onset within 2 min, duration 30–60 min (longer with epi). Amide group. Use "cardiac lidocaine" (ie, IV formulation) for Bier blocks at max dose of 3 mg/kg so that neither epinephrine nor methylparaben is injected IV.

MOA – Amide local anesthetic.

ADVERSE EFFECTS – Serious: Seizures, cardiovascular depression, bradycardia, hypersensitivity, methemoglobinemia. Frequent: None.

[14] CHLOROPROCAINE (*Nesacaine*)

▶LK ♀C ▶? $

ADULT – Epidural anesthesia: 18–24 mL of 2.0–3.0% chloroprocaine will provide 30–60 min of surgical anesthesia. Infiltration and peripheral nerve block: 0.5–40 mL of 1%-3% chloroprocaine.

PEDS – Same as adult, age 3 yo or older.

FORMS – 1, 2, 3%.

NOTES – Max local dose: 11 mg/kg.

MOA – Ester local anesthetic.

ADVERSE EFFECTS – Serious: Seizures, cardiovascular depression, bradycardia, hypersensitivity, methemoglobinemia. Frequent: None.

[15]ROPIVACAINE *(Naropin)*

▶LK ♀B ▶? $

WARNING – Inadvertent intravascular injection may result in arrhythmia or cardiac arrest.

ADULT – Local and regional anesthesia: 0.2–1% injection.

PEDS – Not approved in children.

FORMS – 0.2, 0.5, 0.75, 1%.

MOA – Amide local anesthetic.

ADVERSE EFFECTS – Serious: Seizures, cardiovascular depression, bradycardia, hypersensitivity, methemoglobinemia. Frequent: None.

[16]KETAMINE *(Ketalar)*

▶L ♀C ▶? ©III $■

WARNING – Postanesthetic emergence reactions up to 24 h later manifested as dreamlike state, vivid imagery, hallucinations, and delirium reported in about 12% of cases. Incidence reduced when (1) age less than 15 yo or greater than 65 yo, (2) concomitant use of benzodiazepines, lower dose, or used as induction agent only (because of use of post-intubation sedation).

ADULT – Induction of anesthesia: Adult: 1–2 mg/kg IV over 1–2 min (produces 5–10 min dissociative state) or 6.5–13 mg/kg IM (produces 10–20 min dissociative state).

PEDS – Age over 16 yo: same as adult.

UNAPPROVED ADULT – Dissociative sedation: 1–2 mg/kg IV over 1–2 mm (sedation lasting 10–20 min); repeat 0.5 mg/kg doses every 5–15 min may be given; 4–5 mg/kg IM (sedation lasting 15–30 min); repeat 2–4 mg/kg IM can be given if needed after 10–15 min. Analgesia adjunct subdissociative dose: 0.01–0.5 mg/kg in conjunction with opioid analgesia.

UNAPPROVED PEDS – Dissociative sedation: Age older than 3 mo: 1–2 mg/kg IV (produces 5–10 min dissociative state) over 1–2 min or 4–5 mg/kg IM (produces 10–20 min dissociative state). Not approved for age younger than 3 mo.

FORMS – Generic/Trade: 10, 50, 100 mg/mL.

NOTES – Recent evidence suggests ketamine is not contraindicated in patients with head injuries. However, avoid if CAD or severe HTN. Concurrent administration of atropine no longer recommended. Consider prophylactic ondansetron to reduce vomiting and prophylactic midazolam (0.3 mg/kg) to reduce recovery reactions.

MOA – NMDA receptor antagonist which produces dissociative state.

ADVERSE EFFECTS – Serious: Laryngospasm, hallucinatory emergence reactions, hypersalivation. Frequent: Nystagmus, hypertension, tachycardia, N/V, muscular hypertonicity, myoclonus.

[17]NITROUS OXIDE *(Entonox)*

▶Respiratory ♀– ▶? Varies

ADULT – General anesthetic gas: Specialized dosing.

PEDS – General anesthetic gas: Specialized dosing.

NOTES – Always maintain at least 20% oxygen administration.

MOA – CNS depressant

ADVERSE EFFECTS – Serious: Apnea, malignant hyperthermia, pressure accumulation (middle ear, bowel obstruction, pneumothorax), abuse dependence. Frequent: Recovery N/V.

[18]DIFLUNISAL *(Dolobid)*

▶K ⊘ ♀C (D in 3rd trimester) ▶–

ADULT – Mild to moderate pain: Initially, 500 mg to 1 g PO, then 250–500 mg PO q8–12h. RA/OA: 500 mg to 1 g PO divided two times per day. Max dose 1.5 g/day.

PEDS – Not approved in children.

FORMS – Generic only: Tabs 500 mg.

NOTES – Do not crush or chew tabs. Increases acetaminophen levels.

MOA – Anti-inflammatory, analgesic.

ADVERSE EFFECTS – Serious: Hypersensitivity, Reye's syndrome, GI bleeding, nephrotoxicity. Frequent: Nausea, dyspepsia.

[19]MORPHINE *(MS Contin, Kadian, Avinza, Roxanol, Oramorph SR, MSIR, DepoDur, Statex, M.O.S. Doloral, M-Eslon)*

▶LK ⊘ ♀C ▶+ ©II Varies by therapy ■

WARNING – Multiple strengths; see FORMS and write specific product on Rx. Drinking alcohol while taking Avinza may result in a rapid release of a potentially fatal dose of morphine.

ADULT – Moderate to severe pain: 10–30 mg PO q4h (immediate-release tabs, or oral soln). Controlled-release (MS Contin, Oramorph SR): 30 mg PO q8–12h (Kadian): 20 mg PO q12–24h. Extended-release caps (Avinza): 30 mg PO daily. 10 mg q4h. IM/SC. 2.5–15 mg/70 kg IV over 4–5 min. 10–20 mg PR q4h. Pain with major surgery (DepoDur): 10–15 mg once epidurally at the lumbar level prior to surgery (max dose 20 mg), or 10 mg epidurally after clamping of the umbilical cord with cesarean section.

PEDS – Moderate to severe pain: 0.1–0.2 mg/kg up to 15 mg IM/SC/IV q2–4h

UNAPPROVED PEDS – Moderate to severe pain: 0.2–0.5 mg/kg/dose PO (immediate-release) q4–6h. 0.3–0.6 mg/kg/dose PO (controlled-release) q12h.

FORMS – Generic only: Tabs, immediate-release 15, 30 mg ($). Oral soln 10 mg/5 mL, 20 mg/5 mL, 20 mg/mL (concentrate). Rectal supps 5, 10, 20, 30 mg. Generic/Trade: Controlled-release tabs (MS Contin) 15, 30, 60, 100, 200 mg ($$$$). Controlled-release caps (Kadian) 10, 20, 30, 50, 60, 80, 100 mg ($$$$$). Extended-release caps (Avinza) 30, 45, 60, 75, 90, 120 mg. Trade only: Controlled-release caps (Kadian) 40, 200 mg.

NOTES – Titrate dose as high as necessary to relieve cancer or nonmalignant pain where chronic opioids are necessary. The active metabolites may accumulate in hepatic/renal insufficiency and the elderly leading to increased analgesic and sedative effects. Do not break, chew, or crush MS Contin or Oramorph SR. Kadian and Avinza caps may be opened and sprinkled in applesauce for easier administration; however, the pellets should not be crushed or chewed. Doses more than 1600 mg/day of Avinza contain a potentially nephrotoxic quantity of fumaric acid. Do not mix DepoDur with other medications; do not administer any other medications into epidural space for at least 48 h. Severe opiate overdose with respiratory depression has occurred with intrathecal leakage of DepoDur.

MOA – Opioid agonist analgesic.

ADVERSE EFFECTS – Serious: Respiratory depression/arrest. Frequent: N/V, constipation, sedation, hypotension.

[20]FENTANYL *(IONSYS, Duragesic, Actiq, Fentora, Sublimaze, Abstral, Subsys, Lazanda, Onsolis)*

▶L ⊗ ♀C ▶+ ©II Varies by therapy ■

WARNING — Duragesic patches, Actiq, Fentora, Abstral, Subsys, and Lazanda are contraindicated in the management of acute or postop pain due to potentially life-threatening respiratory depression in opioid nontolerant patients. Instruct patients and their caregivers that even used patches/lozenges on a stick can be fatal to a child or pet. Dispose via toilet. Actiq and Fentora are not interchangeable. IONSYS: For hospital use only; remove prior to discharge. Can cause life-threatening respiratory depression.

ADULT — Duragesic patches: Chronic pain: 12–100 mcg/h patch q72h. Titrate dose to the needs of the patient. Some patients require q48h dosing. May wear more than 1 patch to achieve the correct analgesic effect. Actiq: Breakthrough cancer pain: 200–1600 mcg sucked over 15 min if 200 mcg ineffective for 6 units use higher strength. Goal is 4 lozenges on a stick/day in conjunction with long-acting opioid. Buccal tab (Fentora) for breakthrough cancer pain: 100–800 mcg, titrated to pain relief; may repeat once after 30 min during single episode of breakthrough pain. See prescribing information for dose conversion from transmucosal lozenges. Buccal soluble film (Onsolis) for breakthrough cancer pain: 200–1200 mcg titrated to pain relief; no more than 4 doses/day separated by at least 2 h. Postop analgesia: 50–100 mcg IM; repeat in 1–2 h prn. SL tab (Abstral) for breakthrough cancer pain: 100 mcg, may repeat once after 30 minutes. Specialized titration. SL spray

(Subsys) for breakthrough cancer pain 100 mcg, may repeat once after 30 minutes. Specialized titration. Nasal spray (Lazanda) for breakthrough cancer pain: 100 mcg. Specialized titration. IONSYS: Acute postop pain: Specialized dosing.

PEDS — Transdermal (Duragesic): Not approved in children younger than 2 yo or in opioid-naïve. Use adult dosing for age older than 2 yo. Children converting to a 25-mcg patch should be receiving 45 mg or more oral morphine equivalents/day. Actiq: Not approved for age younger than 16 yo. IONSYS not approved in children. Abstral, Subsys, and Lazanda: Not approved for age younger than 18.

UNAPPROVED ADULT — Analgesia/procedural sedation/labor analgesia: 50–100 mcg IV or IM q1–2h prn.

UNAPPROVED PEDS — Analgesia: 1–2 mcg/kg/dose IV/IM q30–60 min prn or continuous IV infusion 1–3 mcg/kg/h (not to exceed adult dosing). Procedural sedation: 2–3 mcg/kg/dose for age 1–3 yo; 1–2 mcg/kg/dose for age 3–12 yo, 0.5–1 mcg/kg/dose (not to exceed adult dosing) for age older than 12 yo, procedural sedation doses may be repeated q30–60 min prn.

FORMS — Generic/Trade: Transdermal patches 12, 25, 50, 75, 100 mcg/h. Actiq lozenges on a stick, berry-flavored 200, 400, 600, 800, 1200, 1600 mcg. Trade only: (Fentora) buccal tab 100, 200, 400, 600, 800 mcg, packs of 4 or 28 tabs. Trade only: (Onsolis) buccal soluble film 200, 400, 600, 800, 1200 mcg in child-resistant, protective foil, packs of 30 films. Trade only: (Abstral) SL tabs 100, 200, 300, 400, 600, 800 mcg, packs of 4 or 32 tabs. Trade only: (Subsys) SL spray 100, 200, 400, 600, 800, 1200, 1600 mcg blister packs in cartons of 10 and

30 (30 only for 1200 and 1600 mcg). Trade only: (Lazanda) nasal spray 100, 400 mcg/spray, 8 sprays/bottle.

NOTES — Do not use patches for acute pain or in opioid-naïve patients. Oral transmucosal fentanyl doses of 5 mcg/kg provide effects similar to 0.75–1.25 mcg/kg of fentanyl IM. Lozenges on a stick should be sucked, not chewed. Flush lozenge remnants (without stick) down the toilet. For transdermal systems: Apply patch to non-hairy skin. Clip (do not shave) hair if you have to apply to hairy area. Fever or external heat sources may increase fentanyl released from patch. Patch should be removed prior to MRI and reapplied after the test. Dispose of a used patch by folding with the adhesive side of the patch adhering to itself then flush it down the toilet immediately. Do not cut the patch in half. For Duragesic patches and Actiq lozenges on a stick: Titrate dose as high as necessary to relieve cancer or nonmalignant pain where chronic opioids are necessary. Do not suck, chew, or swallow buccal tab. IONSYS: Apply to intact skin on the chest or upper arm. Each dose activated by the patient is delivered over a 10-min period. Remove prior to hospital discharge. Do not allow gel to touch mucous membranes. Dispose using gloves. Keep all forms of fentanyl out of the reach of children or pets. Concomitant use with potent CYP3A4 inhibitors such as ritonavir, ketoconazole, itraconazole, clarithromycin, nelfinavir, and nefazodone may result in an increase in fentanyl plasma concentrations, which could increase or prolong adverse drug effects and may cause potentially fatal respiratory depression. Onsolis is available only through the FOCUS Program and requires prescriber, pharmacy, and patient enrollment. Used films should be discarded into

toilet. Abstral, Subsys, and Lazanda: Outpatients, prescribers, pharmacies, and distributors must be enrolled in TIRF REMS Access program before patient may receive medication.
MOA – Opioid agonist analgesic.
ADVERSE EFFECTS – Serious: Respiratory depression/arrest, chest wall rigidity. Frequent: N/V, constipation, sedation, skin irritation, dental decay with Actiq.

[21]HYDROMORPHONE *(Dilaudid, Exalgo, Hydromorph Contin)*

▶L ⊗ ♀C ▷? ©II $$■

ADULT – Moderate to severe pain: 2–4 mg PO q4–6h. Initial dose (opioid-naïve): 0.5–2 mg SC/IM or slow IV q4–6h prn. 3 mg PR q6–8h. Controlled-release tabs: 8–64 mg daily.
PEDS – Not approved in children.
UNAPPROVED PEDS – Pain age 12 yo or younger: 0.03–0.08 mg/kg PO q4–6h prn. 0.015 mg/kg/dose IV q4–6h prn, use adult dose for older than 12 yo.
FORMS – Generic/Trade: Tabs 2, 4, 8 mg (8 mg trade scored). Oral soln 5 mg/5 mL. Controlled-release tabs (Exalgo): 8, 12, 16, 32 mg.
NOTES – In opioid-naïve patients, consider an initial dose of 0.5 mg or less IM/SC/IV. SC/IM/IV doses after initial dose should be individualized. May be given by slow IV injection over 2–5 min. Titrate dose as high as necessary to relieve cancer or nonmalignant pain where chronic opioids are necessary. 1.5 mg IV = 7.5 mg PO. Exalgo intended for opioid-tolerant patients only.
MOA – Opioid agonist analgesic.
ADVERSE EFFECTS – Serious: Respiratory depression/arrest. Frequent: N/V, constipation, sedation.

[22]SUFENTANIL *(Sufenta)*

▶L ♀C ▶? ©II $$

ADULT – General anesthesia: Induction: 8–30 mcg/kg IV; maintenance 0.5–10 mcg/kg IV. Conscious sedation: Loading dose: 0.1–0.5 mcg/kg; maintenance infusion 0.005–0.01 mcg/kg/min.

PEDS – General anesthesia: Induction: 8–30 mcg/kg IV; maintenance 0.5–10 mcg/kg IV. Conscious sedation: Loading dose: 0.1–0.5 mcg/kg; maintenance infusion 0.005–0.01 mcg/kg/min.

MOA – Serious: Respiratory depression, hypotension, bradycardia, chest wall rigidity, opiate dependence, hypersensitivity. Frequent: Sedation, N/V.

[23]NORCO *(hydrocodone + acetaminophen)*

▶L ⊗ ♀C ▶? ©II $$

WARNING – Multiple strengths; see FORMS and write specific product on Rx.

ADULT – Moderate to severe pain: 1–2 tabs PO q4–6h prn (5/325), max dose 12 tabs/day. 1 tab (7.5/325 and 10/325) PO q4–6h prn, max dose 8 and 6 tabs/day, respectively.

PEDS – Not approved in children.

FORMS – Generic/Trade: Tabs 5/325, 7.5/325, 10/325 mg hydrocodone/acetaminophen, scored. Generic only: Soln 7.5/325 mg per 15 mL.

[24]VICODIN *(hydrocodone + acetaminophen)*

▶LK ⊗ ♀C ▶? ©II $$$

WARNING – Multiple strengths; see FORMS and write specific product on Rx.

ADULT – Moderate pain: 5/300 mg (max dose 8 tabs/day) and 7.5/300 mg (max dose of 6 tabs/day): 1–2 tabs PO q4–6h prn. 10/300 mg: 1 tab PO q4–6h prn (max of 6 tabs/day).
PEDS – Not approved in children.
FORMS – Generic/Trade: Tabs Vicodin (5/300), Vicodin ES (7.5/300), Vicodin HP (10/300) mg hydrocodone/mg acetaminophen, scored.

[24]LORTAB (hydrocodone + acetaminophen)

▶LK ✪ ♀C ▶– ©II $$
WARNING – Multiple strengths; see FORMS and write specific product on Rx.
ADULT – Moderate pain: 1–2 tabs 2.5/325 and 5/325 PO q4–6h prn, max dose 8 tabs/day. 1 tab 7.5/325 and 10/325 PO q4–6h prn, max dose 5 tabs/day.
PEDS – Not approved in children.
FORMS – Generic/Trade: Lortab 5/325 (scored), Lortab 7.5/325 (trade scored), Lortab 10/325 mg hydrocodone/mg acetaminophen. Generic only: Tabs 2.5/325 mg.
MOA – Serious: Respiratory depression/arrest, hepatotoxicity. Frequent: N/V, constipation, sedation.

[24]LORCET (hydrocodone + acetaminophen)

▶LK ✪ ♀C ▶– ©II $$
WARNING – Multiple strengths; see FORMS and write specific product on Rx.
ADULT – Moderate pain: 1–2 caps (5/325) PO q4–6h prn, max dose 8 caps/day. 1 tab PO q4–6h prn (7.5/325 and 10/325), max dose 6 tabs/day.
PEDS – Not approved in children.
FORMS – Generic/Trade: Tabs, 5/325, 7.5/325,10/325 mg.

[25]VICOPROFEN *(hydrocodone + ibuprofen)*

▶LK ❷♀–▶? ⊙ll $$

ADULT – Moderate pain: 1 tab PO q4–6h prn, max dose 5 tabs/day.

PEDS – Not approved in children.

FORMS – Generic/Trade: Tabs 7.5/200 mg hydrocodone/ ibuprofen. Generic only: Tabs 2.5/200, 5/200, 10/200 mg.

NOTES – See NSAIDs: Other subclass warning.

MOA – Combination analgesic.

ADVERSE EFFECTS – Serious: Respiratory depression/arrest, hypersensitivity, GI bleeding, nephrotoxicity. Frequent: N/V, constipation, dyspepsia, sedation.

[26] PERCOCET *(oxycodone + acetaminophen, Percocet-Demi, Oxycocet, Endocet)*

▶L ❷♀C▶– ⊙ll $

WARNING – Multiple strengths; see FORMS and write specific product on Rx.

ADULT – Moderate to severe pain: 1–2 tabs PO q4–6h prn (2.5/325 and 5/325 mg). 1 tab PO q4–6h prn (7.5/325 and 10/325 mg).

PEDS – Not approved in children.

FORMS – Generic/Trade: Oxycodone/acetaminophen tabs 2.5/325, 5/325, 7.5/325, 10/325 mg. Trade only: (Primlev) tabs 2.5/300, 5/300, 7.5/300, 10/300 mg. Generic only: 10/325 mg.

[26] ROXICET *(oxycodone + acetaminophen)*

▶L ❷♀C▶– ⊙ll $

WARNING – Multiple strengths; see FORMS and write specific product on Rx.

MUSCULOSKELETAL PAIN (Traumatic/Non-Traumatic)

ADULT — Moderate to severe pain: 1 tab PO q6h prn. Oral soln: 5 mL PO q6h prn.

PEDS — Not approved in children.

FORMS — Generic/Trade: Tabs 5/325 mg. Caps/caplets 5/325 mg. Soln 5/325 per 5 mL mg oxycodone/acetaminophen.

NEUROPATHIC PAIN (INCLUDING RADICULAR BACK PAIN)

Inpatient Analgesics (in the ED)	Outpatient Analgesics (discharge)
Non-Opioid	**Non-Opioid**

<table>
<tr>
<td>

Oral Analgesics:
[1]**Ibuprofen:** 400 mg, or
[2]**Naproxen:** 500 mg, or
[3]**Diclofenac:** 50 mg, or
[4]**Ketorolac:** 10 mg.
[5]**Acetaminophen:** 500 mg, best if combined with ibuprofen 400 mg or naproxen 500 mg.
[6]**Gabapentin:** 100 mg.
[7]**Pregabalin:** 25 mg.
[8]**Lidocaine:** 5% patch (apply to affected area up to 3 patches per day).

Parenteral Regimen:
[9]**Ketamine (Subdissociative Dose, SDK)**

- **IV:** 0.3 mg/kg over 15 min, +/− continuous IV infusion at 0.15–0.2 mg/kg/h
- **SQ:** 0.3 mg/kg over 15 min, +/− continuous SQ infusion at 0.15–0.2 mg/kg/h

</td>
<td>

[1]**PO Ibuprofen:** 400 mg q8h × 3 days (max 5 days with 1200 mg/d).

[5]**PO Acetaminophen:** 500 mg PO q8h × 3 days (max 1500 mg/day). Best if combined with [1]**Ibuprofen** at 400 mg q8h.

[16]**PO Diflunisal** (Dolobid): 250–500 mg PO q12h × 3 days.

[2]**PO Naproxen:** 500 mg q12h × 3 days (max 5 days).

[3]**PO Diclofenac:** 50 mg q8h × 3 days (max 5 days).

[6]**PO Gabapentin:** 100 mg q8h (titrate by 100 mg every other day up to 600–900 mg/day).

</td>
</tr>
</table>

(continues)

Inpatient Analgesics (in the ED)	Outpatient Analgesics (discharge)
Non-Opioid	**Non-Opioid**
• **Intranasal (IN):** 0.5–1 mg/kg (weight-based) q5–10 min (consider using highly concentrated solutions: Adults: 100 mg/mL; Peds: 50 mg/mL. No more than 0.3–0.5 mL/per nostril), and titrate to the effect.	[7]**PO Pregabalin:** 25 mg q8h (titrate by 25 mg every other day up to 150 mg/day).
[10]**IV Magnesium:** 1 g over 30–45 min (as adjunct to ketamine).	[17]**Topical Diclofenac Gel/Patch:** Apply thin layer to affected area q12h for 5–7 days; apply patch to affected area q12h for 5–7 days.
[11]**IV Lidocaine:** 1.5 mg/kg of 2% (preservative-free lidocaine-cardiac or pre-made bags only) over 10–15 min (max dose 200 mg) + continuous infusion at 1.5–2.5 mg/kg/h.	[8]**Topical Lidocaine** (2% cream): apply thin layer to affected area q12h × 5–7 days.
[12]**IV Dexmedetomidine:** 0.5–1 µg/kg over 10–15 min (bolus); 0.1–0.2 µg/kg/h continuous infusion (range 0.1–1 µg/kg/h) with titration as needed.	[8]**Topical Lidoderm** (4–5% patch): 2 patches max for 12h on skin, then 12h patch-free period × 5–7 days.
[13]**IV Clonidine:** 1.5–3.0 µg/kg over 10–15 min (bolus); 0.1–0.3 µg/kg/h continuous infusion with titration as needed.	[18]**Topical Capsaicin** (0.025–0.15% cream): apply q12h to affected area × 5–7 days. Avoid contact with mucous membranes.

(*continues*)

Inpatient Analgesics (in the ED)	Outpatient Analgesics (discharge)
Non-Opioid	Non-Opioid
<u>Regional Block for Acute Herpetic Neuralgia (cervico-facial, thoracic, or abdominal distribution):</u> [14]**Bupivacaine** w/o epi: 0.25–0.5%, max 2.5 mg/kg. [14]**Bupivacaine** with epi: 0.25–0.5%, max 3.0 mg/kg. [11]**Lidocaine** w/o epi: 0.5–2%, 4.5 mg/kg, max 300 mg. [11]**Lidocaine** with epi: 0.5–2%, 7 mg/kg, max 500 mg. [15]**Chloroprocaine** 2–3%, max 11 mg/kg.	

[1]**IBUPROFEN** *(Motrin, Advil, Nuprin, Rufen, NeoProfen, Caldolor)*

▶L ⊘ ♀B (D in 3rd trimester) ▶+ ■

ADULT — RA/OA, gout: 200–800 mg PO three to four times per day. Mild to moderate pain: 400 mg PO q4–6h; 400–800 mg IV (Caldolor) q6h prn; 400 mg IV (Caldolor) q4–6h or 100–200 mg q4h prn. Primary dysmenorrhea: 400 mg PO q4h prn. Fever: 200 mg PO q4–6h prn. Migraine pain: 200–400 mg PO not to exceed 400 mg in 24 h unless directed by a physician (OTC dosing). Max dose 3.2 g/day.

PEDS — JRA: 30–50 mg/kg/day PO divided qGh. Max dose 2400 mg/24 h. 20 mg/kg/day may be adequate for milder disease. Analgesic/antipyretic, age older than 6 mo: 5–10 mg/kg PO q6 to 8 h, prn. Max dose 40 mg/kg/day. Patent ductus arteriosus in neonates 32 weeks' gestational age or younger weighing 500–1500 g (NeoProfen): Specialized dosing.

FORMS — OTC: Caps/Liqui-Gel caps 200 mg. Tabs 100, 200 mg. Chewable tabs 100 mg. Susp (infant gtts) 50 mg/1.25 mL (with calibrated dropper), 100 mg/5 mL. Rx Generic/Trade: Tabs 400, 600, 800 mg.

NOTES — May antagonize antiplatelet effects of aspirin if given simultaneously. Take aspirin 2 h prior to ibuprofen. Administer IV (Caldolor) over at least 30 min; hydration important.

MOA — Anti-inflammatory/antipyretic, analgesic.

ADVERSE EFFECTS — Serious: Hypersensitivity, GI bleeding, nephrotoxicity. Frequent: Nausea, dyspepsia.

[2]NAPROXEN *(Naprosyn, Aleve, Anaprox, EC-Naprosyn, Naprelan, Prevacid, NapraPAC)*

▶L ✪ ♀B (D in 3rd trimester) ▶+ $■

WARNING — Multiple strengths; see FORMS and write specific product on Rx.

ADULT — RA/OA, ankylosing spondylitis, pain, dysmenorrhea, acute tendinitis and bursitis, fever: 250–500 mg PO two times per day. Delayed-release: 375–500 mg PO two times per day (do not crush or chew). Controlled-release: 750–1000 mg PO daily. Acute gout: 750 mg PO once, then 250 mg PO q8h until the attack subsides. Controlled-release: 1000–1500 mg PO once, then 1000 mg PO daily until the attack subsides.

PEDS – JRA: 10–20 mg/kg/day PO divided two times per day (up to 1250 mg/24 h). Pain for age older than 2 yo: 5–7 mg/kg/dose PO q8–12 h.

UNAPPROVED ADULT – Acute migraine: 750 mg PO once, then 250–500 mg PO prn. Migraine prophylaxis, menstrual migraine: 500 mg PO two times per day beginning 1 day prior to onset of menses and ending on last day of period.

FORMS – OTC Generic/Trade (Aleve): Tabs, immediate-release 200 mg. OTC Trade only (Aleve): Caps, Gelcaps, immediate-release 200 mg. Rx Generic/Trade: Tabs, immediate-release (Naprosyn) 250, 375, 500 mg. (Anaprox) 275, 550 mg. Tabs, delayed-release enteric-coated (EC-Naprosyn) 375, 500 mg. Tabs, controlled-release (Naprelan) 375, 500, 750 mg. Susp (Naprosyn) 125 mg/5 mL. Prevacid NapraPAC: 7 lansoprazole 15 mg caps packaged with 14 naproxen tabs 375 mg or 500 mg.

NOTES – All dosing is based on naproxen content: 500 mg naproxen is equivalent to 550 mg naproxen sodium.

MOA – Anti-inflammatory, analgesic.

ADVERSE EFFECTS – Serious: Hypersensitivity, GI bleeding, nephrotoxicity. Frequent: Nausea, dyspepsia.

[3]DICLOFENAC *(Voltaren, Voltaren XR, Flector, Zipsor, Cambia, Zorvolex, Voltaren Rapide)*

▶L ⊗ ♀B (D in 3rd trimester) ▶– $$$■

WARNING – Multiple strengths; see FORMS and write specific product on Rx.

ADULT – OA: Immediate- or delayed-release: 50 mg PO two to three times per day or 75 mg two times per day.

Extended-release 100 mg PO daily. Gel: Apply 4 g to knees or 2 g to hands four times per day using enclosed dosing card. RA: Immediate- or delayed-release 50 mg PO three to four times per day or 75 mg two times per day. Extended-release 100 mg PO one to two times per day. Ankylosing spondylitis: Immediate- or delayed-release 25 mg PO four times per day and at bedtime. Analgesia and primary dysmenorrhea: Immediate- or delayed release 50 mg PO three times per day. Acute pain in strains, sprains, or contusions: Apply 1 patch to painful area two times per day. Acute migraine with or without aura: 50 mg single dose (Cambia), mix packet with 30–60 mL water.

PEDS – Not approved in children.

UNAPPROVED PEDS – JRA: 2–3 mg/kg/day PO.

FORMS – Generic/Trade: Tabs, extended-release (Voltaren XR) 100 mg. Topical gel (Voltaren) 1% 100 g tube. Generic only: Tabs, immediate-release: 25, 50 mg. Generic only: Tabs, delayed-release: 25, 50, 75 mg. Trade only: Patch (Flector) 1.3% diclofenac epolamine. Trade only: Caps, liquid-filled (Zipsor) 25 mg. Caps (Zorvolex) 18, 35 mg. Trade only: Powder for oral soln (Cambia) 50 mg.

NOTES – Check LFTs at baseline, within 4–8 weeks of initiation, then periodically. Do not apply patch to damaged or nonintact skin. Wash hands, and avoid eye contact when handling the patch. Do not wear patch while bathing or showering.

MOA – Anti-inflammatory, analgesic.

ADVERSE EFFECTS – Serious: Hypersensitivity, GI bleeding, hepato/nephrotoxicity. Frequent: Nausea, dyspepsia, pruritus and dermatitis with patch and gel.

[4]KETOROLAC *(Toradol)*

▶L ⊗ ♀B (D in 3rd trimester) ▶+ $$ ■

WARNING – Indicated for short-term (up to 5 days) therapy only. Ketorolac is a potent NSAID and can cause serious GI and renal adverse effects. It may also increase the risk of bleeding by inhibiting platelet function. Contraindicated in patients with active peptic ulcer disease, recent GI bleeding or perforation, a history of peptic ulcer disease or GI bleeding, or advanced renal impairment.

ADULT – Moderately severe, acute pain, single-dose treatment: 30–60 mg IM or 15–30 mg IV. Multiple-dose treatment: 15–30 mg IV/IM q6h. IV/IM doses are not to exceed 60 mg/day for age 65 yo or older, wt < 50 kg, and patients with moderately elevated serum creatinine. Oral continuation therapy: 10 mg PO q4–6h prn, max dose 40 mg/day. Combined duration IV/IM and PO is not to exceed 5 days.

PEDS – Not approved in children.

UNAPPROVED PEDS – Pain: 0.5 mg/kg/dose IM/IV q6h (up to 30 mg q6h or 120 mg/day), give 10 mg PO qGh pm (up to 40 mg/day) for wt > 50 kg.

FORMS – Generic only: Tabs 10 mg.

MOA – Serious: Hypersensitivity, GI bleeding, nephrotoxicity. Frequent: Nausea, dyspepsia.

[5]ACETAMINOPHEN *(Tylenol, Panadol, Tempra, Ofirmev, Paracetamol, Abenol, Atasol, Pediatrix)*

▶LK ♀B ▶+ $

ADULT – Analgesic/antipyretic: 325–1000 mg PO q4–6h pm. 650 mg PR q4–6h pm. Max dose 4 g/day. OA: Extended-release: 2 caps PO q8h around the clock. Max dose 6 caps/day.

PEDS — Analgesic/antipyretic: 10–15 mg/kg q4–6h PO/PR pm. Max 5 doses/day.

UNAPPROVED ADULT — OA: 1000 mg PO four times per day.

FORMS — OTC: Tabs 325, 500, 650 mg. Chewable tabs 80 mg. Orally disintegrating tabs 80, 160 mg. Caps/gelcaps 500 mg. Extended-release caplets 650 mg. Liquid 160 mg/5 mL, 500 mg/15 mL. Supps 80, 120, 325, 650 mg.

[6] GABAPENTIN *(Neurontin, Horizant, Gralise)*

▶K ⊗ ♀C ▶? $$$$

ADULT — Partial seizures, adjunctive therapy: Start 300 mg PO three times daily. Gradually increase to recommended dose of 300–600 mg PO three times per day. Doses of up to 2400 mg/day have been well tolerated. Max 3600 mg/day divided three times per day. Post-herpetic neuralgia, immediate-release tabs: Start 300 mg PO on day 1; increase to 300 mg two times per day on day 2, and to 300 mg three times per day on day 3. Usual maintenance dose 1800 mg/day divided three times per day. Doses as high as 3600 mg/day have been used but are not more effective. Post-herpetic neuralgia (Gralise): Start 300 mg PO once daily with evening meal. Increase to 600 mg on day 2, 900 mg on days 3 to 6, 1200 mg on days 7 to 10, 1500 mg on days 11–14, and 1800 mg on day 15. Max 1800 mg/day. Post-herpetic neuralgia (Horizant): Start 600 mg PO qam for 3 days, then increase to 600 mg PO twice per day. Max 1200 mg/day. Restless legs syndrome (Horizant): 600 mg PO once daily around 5 PM taken with food.

PEDS — Partial seizures, adjunctive therapy: Start 10–15 mg/kg/day PO divided three times per day for age 3 to 11 yo. Titrate over 3 days to recommended dose of 40 mg/kg/day (3 yo to 4 yo) or 25 mg/kg/day to 35 mg/kg/day (5 yo to 11 yo). Give in 3 divided doses. Use adult dosing for age 12 yo and older.

UNAPPROVED ADULT — Neuropathic pain: 300 mg PO three times per day, max 3600/day in 3 to 4 divided doses. Migraine prophylaxis: Start 300 mg PO daily, then gradually increase to 1200–2400 mg/day in 3 to 4 divided doses. Restless legs syndrome: Start 300 mg PO at bedtime. Max 3600 mg/day divided three times per day. Hot flashes: 300 mg PO three times per day.

UNAPPROVED PEDS — Neuropathic pain: Start 5 mg/kg PO at bedtime. Increase to 5 mg/kg twice per day on day 2 and 5 mg/kg three times per day on day 3. Titrate to usual effective level of 8–35 mg/kg/24 h.

FORMS — Generic/ only: Tabs 100, 300, 400 mg. Generic/ Trade: Caps 100, 300, 400 mg. Tabs 100, 300, 400, 600, 800 mg. Soln 50 mg/mL. Trade only: Tabs, extended-release 300, 600 mg (gabapentin enacarbil, Horizant). Trade only (Gralise): Tabs 300, 600 mg.

NOTES — Reduce dose in renal impairment (CrCl < 60 mL/min); Refer to package label for details and prescribing information. Discontinue gradually over 1 week or longer. Do not substitute other brands for Gralise because of bioavailability differences.

MOA — Unknown. Does not appear to be a GABA analogue.

ADVERSE EFFECTS — Serious: Leukopenia, rhabdomyolysis. Frequent: Fatigue, drowsiness, dizziness, ataxia, nystagmus, tremor, peripheral edema, weight gain, suicidality. Peds only: Emotional lability, hostility, hyperactivity.

[7] PREGABALIN *(Luminal)*

▶K ⊗ ♀?/?/?R Evidence teratogenicity in animals. Inadequate human data. Enroll in registry; refer to prescribing information ▶? ©V $$$$$

ADULT – Painful diabetic peripheral neuropathy: Start 50 mg PO three times per day; may increase within 1 week to max 100 mg PO three times per day. Post-herpetic neuralgia: Start 150 mg/day PO divided two to three times per day. May increase within 1 week to 300 mg/day divided two to three times per day. If needed and tolerated, may increase to 600 mg/day in two to three divided doses. Partial seizures (adjunctive): Start 75 mg PO twice daily or 50 mg PO three times daily. Increase as needed to max 600 mg/day. Fibromyalgia: Start 75 mg PO two times per day; may increase to 150 mg two times per day within 1 week; max 225 mg two times per day. Neuropathic pain associated with spinal cord injury: Start 75 mg PO two times per day; may increase to 150 mg two times per day within 1 week and then to 300 mg two times per day after 2–3 weeks if needed and tolerated.

PEDS – Not approved in children.

FORMS – Trade only: Caps 25, 50, 75, 100, 150, 200, 225, 300 mg. Oral soln 20 mg/mL (480 mL).

NOTES – Adjust dose if CrCl less than 60 mL/min; refer to prescribing information. Warn patients to report changes in visual acuity and muscle pain. May increase creative kinase. Must taper if discontinuing to avoid withdrawal symptoms. Increased risk or peripheral edema when used in conjunction with thiazolidinedione antidiabetic agents.

MOA – Unknown. Binds to alpha-2–delta subunit of voltage-gated calcium channels and reduced neurotransmitter release.

ADVERSE EFFECTS – Serious: Angioedema, visual field changes, reduced visual acuity, thrombocytopenia, suicidality, peripheral edema. Frequent: Dizziness, somnolence, dry mouth, decreased concentration/attention, blurred vision, peripheral edema, weight gain, ataxia, withdrawal reactions.

[8]LIDOCAINE—TOPICAL (Xylocaine, Lidoderm, Numby Stuff, LMX, Zingo, Maxilene)

▶LK ♀B ▶+ $

WARNING – Contraindicated in allergy to amide-type anesthetics.

ADULT – Topical anesthesia: Apply to affected area prn. Dose varies with anesthetic procedure, degree of anesthesia required, and individual patient response. Post-herpetic neuralgia (patch): Apply up to 3 patches to affected area at once for up to 12 h within a 24 h period.

PEDS – Topical anesthesia: Apply to affected area prn. Dose varies with anesthetic procedure, degree of anesthesia required, and individual patient response. Max 3 mg/kg/dose, do not repeat dose within 2 h. Intradermal powder injection for venipuncture/IV cannulation, for age 3 to 18 yo (Zingo): 0.5 mg to site 1–10 min prior.

UNAPPROVED PEDS – Topical anesthesia prior to venipuncture: Apply 30 min prior to procedure (ELA-Max 4%).

FORMS – For membranes of mouth and pharynx: Spray 10%, oint 5%, liquid 5%, soln 2%, 4% dental patch. For urethral use: Jelly 2%. Patch (Lidoderm $$$$$) 5%. Intradermal powder injection system: 0.5 mg (Zingo). OTC Trade only: Liposomal lidocaine 4% (ELA-Max).

NOTES — Apply patches only to intact skin to cover the most painful area. Patches may be cut into smaller sizes with scissors prior to removal of the release liner. Store and dispose out of the reach of children and pets to avoid possible toxicity from ingestion.

MOA — Anesthetic.

ADVERSE EFFECTS — Frequent: Skin irritation. Severe: CNS effects, bradycardia, bronchospasm, hypotension, allergic reactions.

[9]KETAMINE *(Ketalar)*

▶L ♀C ▶? ©III $■■

WARNING — Postanesthetic emergence reactions up to 24 h later manifested as dreamlike state, vivid imagery, hallucinations, and delirium reported in about 12% of cases. Incidence reduced when (1) age less than 15 yo or greater than 65 yo, (2) concomitant use of benzodiazepines, lower dose, or used as induction agent only (because of use of post-intubation sedation).

ADULT — Induction of anesthesia: Adult: 1–2 mg/kg IV over 1–2 min (produces 5–10 min dissociative state) or 6.5–13 mg/kg IM (produces 10–20 min dissociative state).

PEDS — Age over 16 yo: same as adult.

UNAPPROVED ADULT — Dissociative sedation: 1–2 mg/kg IV over 1–2 mm (sedation lasting 10–20 min); repeat 0.5 mg/kg doses every 5–15 min may be given; 4–5 mg/kg IM (sedation lasting 15–30 min); repeat 2–4 mg/kg IM can be given if needed after 10–15 min. Analgesia adjunct subdissociative dose: 0.01–0.5 mg/kg in conjunction with opioid analgesia.

UNAPPROVED PEDS — Dissociative sedation: Age older than 3 mo: 1–2 mg/kg IV (produces 5–10 min dissociative state) over

1–2 min or 4–5 mg/kg IM (produces 10–20 min dissociative state). Not approved for age younger than 3 mo.

FORMS – Generic/Trade: 10, 50, 100 mg/mL.

NOTES – Recent evidence suggests ketamine is not contra-indicated in patients with head injuries. However, avoid if CAD or severe HTN. Concurrent administration of atropine no longer recommended. Consider prophylactic ondansetron to reduce vomiting and prophylactic midazolam (0.3 mg/kg) to reduce recovery reactions.

MOA – NMDA receptor antagonist which produces dissociative state.

ADVERSE EFFECTS – Serious: Laryngospasm, hallucinatory emergence reactions, hypersalivation. Frequent: Nystagmus, hypertension, tachycardia, N/V, muscular hypertonicity, myoclonus.

[10]MAGNESIUM SULFATE

▶K ♀D C/D ▶+ $

ADULT – Hypomagnesemia: Mild deficiency: 1 g IM q6h for 4 doses; severe deficiency: 2 g IV over 1 h (monitor for hypotension). Hyperalimentation: Maintenance requirements not precisely known; adults generally require 8–24 mEq/day. Seizure prevention in severe preeclampsia or eclampsia: ACOG recommendations: 4–6 g IV loading dose then 1–2 g/h IV continuous infusion for at least 24 h. Or per product information: Total initial dose of 10–14 g administered via IV infusion and IM doses (4 g IV infusion with 5 g IM injections in each buttock). Initial dose is followed by 4–5 g IM into alternate buttocks q4h prn or initial dose is followed by 1–2 g/h constant IV infusion. Max: 30–40 g/24 h.

PEDS – Not approved in children.

UNAPPROVED ADULT — Preterm labor: 6 g IV over 20 min, then 1–3 g/h titrated to decrease contractions. Has been used as an adjunctive bronchodilator in very severe acute asthma (2 g IV over 10–20 min), and in chronic fatigue syndrome. Torsades de pointes: 1–2 g IV in D5W over 5–60 min.

UNAPPROVED PEDS — Hypomagnesemia: 25–50 mg/kg IV/IM q4–6h for 3 to 4 doses, max single dose 2 g. Hyperalimentation: Maintenance requirements not precisely known; infants require 2–10 mEq/day. Acute nephritis: 20–40 mg/kg (in 20% soln) IM prn. Adjunctive bronchodilator in very severe acute asthma: 25–100 mg/kg IV over 10–20 min.

NOTES — 1000 mg magnesium sulfate contains 8 mEq elem magnesium. Do not give faster than 1.5 mL/min (of 10% soln) except in eclampsia or seizures. Use caution in renal insufflciency, may accumulate. Monitor urine output, patellar reflex, repiratory rate, and serum magnesium level. Concomitant use with terbutaline may lead to fatal pulmonary edema. IM administration must be diluted to a 20% soln. If needed may reverse toxicity with calcium gluconate 1 g IV. Continuous use in pregnancy beyond 5–7 days may cause fetal harm.

MOA — Essential mineral needed for muscle function, organ function, potassium and calcium absorption; blocks neuromuscular transmission to prevent or control convulsions.

ADVERSE EFFECTS — Serious: Magnesium intoxication (in recipient of drug or in newborn of pregnant woman receiving Mg), cardiac depression, respiratory paralysis, hypotension, stupor, hypothermia, circulatory collapse. Frequent: Flushing, sweating, depressed reflexes.

[11]LIDOCAINE—LOCAL ANESTHETIC *(Xylocaine)*

▶LK ♀B ▶? $

ADULT – Without epinephrine: Max dose 4.5 mg/kg not to exceed 300 mg. With epinephrine: Max dose 7 mg/kg not to exceed 500 mg. Dose for regional block varies by region.

PEDS – Same as adult.

FORMS – 0.5, 1, 1.5, 2%. With epi: 0.5, 1, 1.5, 2%.

NOTES – Onset within 2 min, duration 30–60 min (longer with epi). Amide group. Use "cardiac lidocaine" (ie, IV formulation) for Bier blocks at max dose of 3 mg/kg so that neither epinephrine nor methylparaben is injected IV.

MOA – Amide local anesthetic.

ADVERSE EFFECTS – Serious: Seizures, cardiovascular depression, bradycardia, hypersensitivity, methemoglobinemia. Frequent: None.

[12]DEXMEDETOMIDINE *(Precedex)*

▶LK ♀C ▶? $$$

ADULT – ICU sedation less than 24 h: Load 1 mcg/kg over 10 min followed by infusion 0.6 mcg/kg/h (ranges from 0.2–1.0 mcg/kg/h) titrated to desired sedation endpoint. Procedural sedation: Load 1 mcg/kg over 10 min followed by infusion of 0.6 mcg/kg/h titrated up or down to clinical effect in range of 0.2–1 mcg/kg/h depending on procedure and patient (0.7 mcg/kg/h for fiberoptic intubation). Reduce dose in impaired hepatic function and geriatric patients.

PEDS – Not recommended age younger than 18 yo.

NOTES – Alpha-2–adrenergic agonist with sedative properties. Beware of bradycardia and hypotension. Avoid in advanced heart block.

MOA – Alpha-2 adrenergic agonist with sedative properties.
ADVERSE EFFECTS – Serious: Bradycardia, heart block, hypotension. Frequent: Sedation.

[13]CLONIDINE-EPIDURAL *(Duraclon)*

▶LK ♀C ▶– $$$$$
WARNING – Not recommended for obstetrical, postpartum, or perioperative pain management due to hypotension and bradycardia. Abrupt discontinuation may result in a rapid BP rise.
ADULT – Severe cancer pain in combination with opioids: Specialized epidural dosing.
PEDS – Severe cancer pain in combination with opioids: Specialized epidural dosing.
NOTES – Bradycardia and hypotension common. May be exacerbated by beta-blockers, certain calcium channel blockers, and digoxin.
MOA – Central analgesic – prevents pain signal transmission to the brain.
ADVERSE EFFECTS – Serious: Bradycardia, hypotension. Frequent: Hypotension, sedation, dry mouth.

[14]BUPIVACAINE *(Marcaine, Sensorcaine)*

▶LK ♀C ▶? $■
ADULT – Local anesthesia, nerve block: 0.25% injection. Up to 2.5 mg/kg without epinephrine and up 3.0 mg/kg with epinephrine.
PEDS – Not recommended in children younger than 12 yo.
FORMS – 0.25%, 0.5%, 0.75%, all with or without epinephrine.
NOTES – Onset 5 min, duration 2–4 h (longer with epi). Amide group.

MOA – Amide local anesthetic.
ADVERSE EFFECTS – Serious: Seizures, cardiovascular depression, bradycardia, hypersensitivity, methemoglobinemia. Frequent: None.

[15]CHLOROPROCAINE *(Nesacaine)*

▶LK ♀C ▶? $
ADULT – Epidural anesthesia: 18–24 mL of 2.0–3.0% chloroprocaine will provide 30–60 min of surgical anesthesia. Infiltration and peripheral nerve block: 0.5–40 mL of 1–3% chloroprocaine.
PEDS – Same as adult, age 3 yo or older.
FORMS – 1, 2, 3%.
NOTES – Max local dose: 11 mg/kg.
MOA – Ester local anesthetic.
ADVERSE EFFECTS – Serious: Seizures, cardiovascular depression, bradycardia, hypersensitivity, methemoglobinemia. Frequent: None.

[16]DIFLUNISAL *(Dolobid)*

▶K ⊗ ♀C (D in 3rd trimester) ▶–
ADULT – Mild to moderate pain: Initially, 500 mg to 1 g PO, then 250–500 mg PO q8–12h. RA/OA: 500 mg to 1 g PO divided two times per day. Max dose 1.5 g/day.
PEDS – Not approved in children.
FORMS – Generic only: Tabs 500 mg.
NOTES – Do not crush or chew tabs. Increases acetaminophen levels.
MOA – Anti-inflammatory, analgesic.

ADVERSE EFFECTS — Serious: Hypersensitivity, Reye's syndrome, GI bleeding, nephrotoxicity. Frequent: Nausea, dyspepsia.

NOTES — Burning occurs in 30% or more of patients but diminishes with continued use. Pain more commonly occurs when applied less than three to four times per day. Wash hands immediately after application.

MOA — Counter-irritant, releases substance P.

ADVERSE EFFECTS — Frequent: Burning, redness, sensation of warmth.

[17]DICLOFENAC-TOPICAL (Solaraze, Voltaren, Pennsaid)

▶LK ♀C Category D at 30 weeks' gestation and beyond. Avoid use starting at 30 weeks' gestation. ▶? $$$

WARNING — Risk of cardiovascular and GI events.

ADULT — Osteoarthritis of areas amenable to topical therapy: 2 g (upper extremities) to 4 g (lower extremities) four times per day (Voltaren). 40 gtts to knee(s) four times daily.

PEDS — Not approved in children.

FORMS — Generic/Trade: Gel 3% (Solaraze) 100 g. Soln 1.5% (Pennsaid) 150 mL. Trade only: Gel 1% (Voltaren) 100 g. Soln 2.0% Pump (Pennsaid) 112 g.

NOTES — Avoid exposure to sun and sunlamps. Use caution in aspirin-sensitive patients. When using for OA (Voltaren), max daily dose 16 g to any single lower extremity joint, 8 g to any single upper extremity joint. Avoid use in setting of aspirin allergy or CABG surgery.

MOA — Inhibits prostaglandins at level of cyclooxygenase.

ADVERSE EFFECTS — Frequent: Rash, abdominal cramps, nausea, indigestion.

[18] CAPSAICIN *(Zostrix, Zostrix-HP, Qutenza)*

▶? ♀? ▶? $

ADULT — Pain due to RA, OA, and neuralgias such as zoster or diabetic neuropathies: Apply to affected area up to three to four times per day. Post-herpetic neuralgia: 1 patch (Qutenza) applied for 1 h in medical office, may repeat every 3 months.

PEDS — Children older than 2 yo: Pain due to RA, OA, and neuralgias such as zoster or diabetic neuropathies: Apply to affected area up to three to four times per day.

UNAPPROVED ADULT — Psoriasis and intractable pruritus, post-mastectomy/post-amputation neuromas (phantom limb pain), vulvar vestibulitis, apocrine chromhidrosis, and reflex sympathetic dystrophy.

FORMS — Rx: Patch 8% (Qutenza). OTC: Generic/Trade: Cream 0.025% 60 g, 0.075% (HP) 60 g. OTC Generic only: Lotion 0.025% 59 mL, 0.075% 59 mL.

RENANL COLIC PAIN

Inpatient Analgesics (in the ED)	Outpatient Analgesics (discharge)
Non-Opioid	**Non-Opioid**
<u>Oral Analgesics (if feasible):</u> [1]**Acetaminophen:** 500 mg, best if combined with NSAIDs. [2]**Ibuprofen:** 400 mg, or [3]**Naproxen:** 500 mg, or [4]**Diclofenac:** 50 mg, or [5]**Ketorolac:** 10 mg. <u>Parenteral Regimen:</u> [5]**IV Ketorolac:** 10–15 mg IVP (analgesic ceiling dose); IM route of ketorolac is discouraged due to pain at injection site, unpredictable absorption, delayed onset of analgesia, and poor response in 25% of patients. [1]**IV Acetaminophen:** 1 g over 15 min (as adjunct to opioid/non-opioid) if patients are NPO/NPR or contraindications to opioids, NSAIDs, lidocaine, or ketamine.	[2]**PO Ibuprofen:** 400 mg q8h × 3 days (max 5 days with 1200 mg/d). [3]**PO Naproxen:** 500 mg q12h × 3 days (max 5 days). [1]**PO Acetaminophen:** 500 mg PO q8h × 3 days (max 1500 mg/day). Best if combined with [2]**Ibuprofen** 400 mg q8h. [4]**PO Diclofenac:** 50 mg q8h × 3 days (max 5 days). [9]**PO Tamsulosin:** 0.4 mg daily until stone passage (only for distal ureteral stones > 6 mm).

(*continues*)

Inpatient Analgesics (in the ED)	Outpatient Analgesics (discharge)
Non-Opioid	**Non-Opioid**
[6]**IV Lidocaine:** 1.5 mg/kg of 2% (preservative-free lidocaine-cardiac or pre-made bags only) over 15 minutes (max dose 200 mg). [7]**Ketamine (Subdissociative Dose, SDK) IV:** 0.3 mg/kg over 10 min, +/− continuous IV infusion at 0.15–0.2 mg/kg/h [8]**IN Desmopressin:** 40 mcg once as adjunct to NSAIDs or ketamine or opioids.	
Opioid	**Opioid**
<u>Oral Regimen:</u> (if feasible) [10]**Morphine:** PO, Morphine Sulfate Immediate Release (MSIR): 15 mg. [11]**Fentanyl:** Transbuccal 100–200 μg dissolvable tablets, repeat at 30-60 min if pain persists. [12]**Hydromorphone:** 2 mg. <u>Parenteral Regimen:</u> [10]**Morphine:** • **IV:** 0.05–0.1mg/kg (weight-based), titrate q10–20 min	**Opioids (for breakthrough pain):** [10]**Morphine Sulfate Immediate Release (MSIR):** 15 mg q6–8h × 2–3 days (opioid-naïve patients). [13]**Hydrocodone/ Acetaminophen (Norco)** 5/325 mg: 1–2 tabs q6–8h × 2–3 days.

(continues)

Inpatient Analgesics (in the ED)	Outpatient Analgesics (discharge)
Opioid	**Opioid**
<ul><li>**IV:** 4–6 mg (fixed), titrate q10–20 min</li><li>**SQ:** 4–6 mg (fixed), re-administer as needed at q30–40 min</li><li>**IM:** 4–6 mg (fixed), re-administer as needed at q30–40 min (IM route should be avoided due to pain upon injection, muscle fibrosis, necrosis, increase in dosing requirements)</li><li>**Nebulized** (via Breath Actuated Nebulizer [BAN]): Adults: 10–20 mg (fixed), repeat q15–20 min up to three doses Peds: 0.2–0.4 mg/kg (weight-based), repeat q15–20 min up to three doses</li><li>**PCA:** Demand dose: 1–2 mg Continuous basal infusion: 0.5–2 mg/h</li></ul>	[14]**Hydrocodone/ Acetaminophen (Vicodin, Lortab, Lorcet) 5/300 mg:** 1–2 tabs q6–8h × 2–3 days. [15]**Hydrocodone/ Ibuprofen (Vicoprofen) 5/200 mg:** 1–2 tabs q6–8h × 2–3 days. [16]**Oxycodone/ Acetaminophen (Percocet, Roxicet) 5/325 mg:** 1–2 tabs q6–8h × 2–3 days. [12]**Hydromorphone:** 2 mg q6–8h × 2–3 days (for opioid-naïve patients start with 2 mg dose).

RENAL COLIC PAIN

(*continues*)

Inpatient Analgesics (in the ED)	Outpatient Analgesics (discharge)
Opioid	Opioid
[11]Fentanyl: • **IV:** 0.25–0.5 µg/kg (weight-based), titrate q10 min • **IV:** 25–50 µg (fixed), titrate q10 min **Nebulized** (via BAN): Adults: 2–4 µg/kg (weight-based), titrate q20–30 min, up to three doses Peds: 2–4 µg/kg (weight-based), titrate q20–30 up to three dose • **Intranasal (IN):** 1–2 µg/kg (weight-based), titrate q5–10 min (consider using highly concentrated solutions: Adults: 100 µg/mL Peds: 50 µg/mL. No more than 0.3–0.5 mL/per nostril) • **Transmucosal:** 15–20 mcg/kg lollipops • **PCA:** Demand dose: 20–50 µg Continuous basal infusion: 0.05 -0.1µg/kg/h	

(continues)

Inpatient Analgesics (in the ED)	Outpatient Analgesics (discharge)
Opioid	Opioid
[12]Hydromorphone: • **IV:** 0.2–0.5 mg initial, titrate q10–15 min • **SQ:** 0.5–1 mg, titrate q30–40 min • **IM:** 0.5–1 mg, titrate q30–40 min (IM route should be avoided due to pain, muscle fibrosis, necrosis, increase in dosing requirements) • **PCA:** Demand dose: 0.2–0.4 mg Continuous basal infusion: 0.1–0.4 mg/h	

[1]**ACETAMINOPHEN** *(Tylenol, Panadol, Tempra, Ofirmev, Paracetamol, Abenol, Atasol, Pediatrix)*
▶LK ♀B ▶+$
ADULT – Analgesic/antipyretic: 325–1000 mg PO q4–6h prn. 650 mg PR q4–6h pm. Max dose 4 g/day. OA: Extended-release: 2 caps PO q8h around the clock. Max dose 6 caps/day.
PEDS – Analgesic/antipyretic: 10–15 mg/kg q4–6h PO/PR pm. Max 5 doses/day.

UNAPPROVED ADULT — OA: 1000 mg PO four times per day.

FORMS — OTC: Tabs 325, 500, 650 mg. Chewable tabs 80 mg. Orally disintegrating tabs 80, 160 mg. Caps/gelcaps 500 mg. Extended-release caplets 650 mg. Liquid 160 mg/5 mL, 500 mg/15 mL. Supps 80, 120, 325, 650 mg.

[2]IBUPROFEN *(Motrin, Advil, Nuprin, Rufen, NeoProfen, Caldolor)*

▶L ☻♀B (D in 3rd trimester) ▶+ ■

ADULT — RA/OA, gout: 200–800 mg PO three to four times per day. Mild to moderate pain: 400 mg PO q4–6h. 400–800 mg IV (Caldolor) q6h prn. 400 mg IV (Caldolor) q4–6h or 100–200 mg q4h prn. Primary dysmenorrhea: 400 mg PO q4h prn. Fever: 200 mg PO q4–6h prn. Migraine pain: 200–400 mg PO not to exceed 400 mg in 24 h unless directed by a physician (OTC dosing). Max dose 3.2 g/day.

PEDS — JRA: 30–50 mg/kg/day PO divided q6h. Max dose 2400 mg/24 h. 20 mg/kg/day may be adequate for milder disease. Analgesic/antipyretic, age older than 6 mo: 5–10 mg/kg PO q6–8h, prn. Max dose 40 mg/kg/day. Patent ductus arteriosus in neonates 32 weeks' gestational age or younger weighing 500–1500 g (NeoProfen): Specialized dosing.

FORMS — OTC: Caps/Liqui-Gel caps 200 mg. Tabs 100, 200 mg. Chewable tabs 100 mg. Susp (infant gtts) 50 mg/1.25 mL (with calibrated dropper), 100 mg/5 mL. Rx Generic/Trade: Tabs 400, 600, 800 mg.

NOTES — May antagonize antiplatelet effects of aspirin if given simultaneously. Take aspirin 2 h prior to ibuprofen. Administer IV (Caldolor) over at least 30 min; hydration important.

MOA — Anti-inflammatory/antipyretic, analgesic.

ADVERSE EFFECTS — Serious: Hypersensitivity, GI bleeding, nephrotoxicity. Frequent: Nausea, dyspepsia.

[3]NAPROXEN *(Naprosyn, Aleve, Anaprox, EC-Naprosyn, Naprelan, Prevacid, NapraPAC)*

▶L ⊗ ♀B (D in 3rd trimester) ▶+ $■

WARNING — Multiple strengths; see FORMS and write specific product on Rx.

ADULT — RA/OA, ankylosing spondylitis, pain, dysmenorrhea, acute tendinitis and bursitis, fever: 250–500 mg PO two times per day. Delayed-release: 375–500 mg PO two times per day (do not crush or chew). Controlled-release: 750–1000 mg PO daily. Acute gout: 750 mg PO once, then 250 mg PO q8h until the attack subsides. Controlled-release: 1000–1500 mg PO once, then 1000 mg PO daily until the attack subsides.

PEDS — JRA: 10–20 mg/kg/day PO divided two times per day (up to 1250 mg/24 h). Pain for age older than 2 yo: 5–7 mg/kg/dose PO q8–12h.

UNAPPROVED ADULT — Acute migraine: 750 mg PO once, then 250–500 mg PO pm. Migraine prophylaxis, menstrual migraine: 500 mg PO two times per day beginning 1 day prior to onset of menses and ending on last day of period.

FORMS — OTC Generic/Trade (Aleve): Tabs, immediate-release 200 mg. OTC Trade only (Aleve): Caps, Gelcaps, immediate-release 200 mg. Rx Generic/Trade: Tabs, immediate-release (Naprosyn) 250, 375, 500 mg. (Anaprox) 275, 550 mg. Tabs, delayed-release enteric-coated (EC-Naprosyn) 375, 500 mg. Tabs, controlled-release (Naprelan) 375, 500, 750 mg. Susp (Naprosyn) 125 mg/5 mL. Prevacid NapraPAC: 7 lansoprazole 15 mg caps packaged with 14 naproxen tabs 375 mg or 500 mg.

NOTES – All dosing is based on naproxen content: 500 mg naproxen is equivalent to 550 mg naproxen sodium.

MOA – Anti-inflammatory, analgesic.

ADVERSE EFFECTS – Serious: Hypersensitivity, GI bleeding, nephrotoxicity. Frequent: Nausea, dyspepsia.

---

[4]DICLOFENAC (Voltaren, Voltaren XR, Flector, Zipsor, Cambia, Zorvolex, Voltaren Rapide)

▶L ⊗ ♀B (D in 3rd trimester) ▶– $$$■

WARNING – Multiple strengths; see FORMS and write specific product on Rx.

ADULT – OA: Immediate- or delayed-release: 50 mg PO two to three times per day or 75 mg two times per day. Extended-release 100 mg PO daily. Gel: Apply 4 g to knees or 2 g to hands four times per day using enclosed dosing card. RA: Immediate- or delayed-release 50 mg PO three to four times per day or 75 mg two times per day. Extended-release 100 mg PO one to two times per day. Ankylosing spondylitis: Immediate- or delayed-release 25 mg PO four times per day and at bedtime. Analgesia and primary dysmenorrhea: Immediate- or delayed-release 50 mg PO three times per day. Acute pain in strains, sprains, or contusions: Apply 1 patch to painful area two times per day. Acute migraine with or without aura: 50 mg single dose (Cambia), mix packet with 30–60 mL water.

PEDS – Not approved in children.

UNAPPROVED PEDS – JRA: 2–3 mg/kg/day PO.

FORMS – Generic/Trade: Tabs, extended-release (Voltaren XR) 100 mg. Topical gel (Voltaren) 1% 100 g tube. Generic only: Tabs, immediate-release: 25, 50 mg. Generic only: Tabs, delayed-release: 25, 50, 75 mg. Trade only: Patch (Flector) 1.3% diclofenac epolamine. Trade only: Caps, liquid-filled (Zipsor) 25 mg. Caps (Zorvolex) 18, 35 mg. Trade only: Powder for oral soln (Cambia) 50 mg.

NOTES – Check LFTs at baseline, within 4–8 weeks of initiation, then periodically. Do not apply patch to damaged or nonintact skin. Wash hands and avoid eye contact when handling the patch. Do not wear patch while bathing or showering.

MOA – Anti-inflammatory, analgesic.

ADVERSE EFFECTS – Serious: Hypersensitivity, GI bleeding, hepato/nephrotoxicity. Frequent: Nausea, dyspepsia, pruritus and dermatitis with patch and gel.

[5]KETOROLAC *(Toradol)*

▶L ❌ ♀B (D in 3rd trimester) ▶+ $$■

WARNING – Indicated for short-term (up to 5 days) therapy only. Ketorolac is a potent NSAID and can cause serious GI and renal adverse effects. It may also increase the risk of bleeding by inhibiting platelet function. Contraindicated in patients with active peptic ulcer disease, recent GI bleeding or perforation, a history of peptic ulcer disease or GI bleeding, or advanced renal impairment.

ADULT – Moderately severe, acute pain, single-dose treatment: 30–60 mg IM or 15–30 mg IV. Multiple-dose treatment: 15–30 mg IV/IM q6h. IV/IM doses are not to exceed 60 mg/day for age 65 yo or older, wt < 50 kg, and patients with moderately elevated serum creatinine. Oral continuation therapy: 1.0 mg PO q4–6h prn, max dose 40 mg/day. Combined duration IV/IM and PO is not to exceed 5 days.

PEDS – Not approved in children.

UNAPPROVED PEDS — Pain: 0.5 mg/kg/dose IM/IV q6h (up to 30 mg q6h or 120 mg/day), give 10 mg PO q6h pm (up to 40 mg/day) for wt > 50 kg.

FORMS — Generic only: Tabs 10 mg.

MOA — Serious: Hypersensitivity, GI bleeding, nephrotoxicity. Frequent: Nausea, dyspepsia.

[6]LIDOCAINE—LOCAL ANESTHETIC *(Xylocaine)*

▶LK ♀B ▶? $

ADULT — Without epinephrine: Max dose 4.5 mg/kg not to exceed 300 mg. With epinephrine: Max dose 7 mg/kg not to exceed 500 mg. Dose for regional block varies by region.

PEDS — Same as adult.

FORMS — 0.5, 1, 1.5, 2%. With epi: 0.5, 1, 1.5, 2%.

NOTES — Onset within 2 min, duration 30–60 min (longer with epi). Amide group. Use "cardiac lidocaine" (ie, IV formulation) for Bier blocks at max dose of 3 mg/kg so that neither epinephrine nor methylparaben are injected IV.

MOA — Amide local anesthetic.

ADVERSE EFFECTS — Serious: Seizures, cardiovascular depression, bradycardia, hypersensitivity, methemoglobinemia. Frequent: None.

[7]KETAMINE *(Ketalar)*

▶L ♀C ▶? ©III $▣

WARNING — Post-anesthetic emergence reactions up to 24 h later manifested as dreamlike state, vivid imagery, hallucinations, and delirium reported in about 12% of cases. Incidence reduced when (1) age less than 15 yo or greater than 65 yo,

(2) concomitant use of benzodiazepines, lower dose, or used as induction agent only (because of use of post-intubation sedation).

ADULT – Induction of anesthesia: Adult: 1–2 mg/kg IV over 1–2 min (produces 5–10 min dissociative state) or 6.5–13 mg/kg IM (produces 10–20 min dissociative state).

PEDS – Age over 16 yo: same as adult.

UNAPPROVED ADULT – Dissociative sedation: 1–2 mg/kg IV over 1–2 mm (sedation lasting 10–20 min); repeat 0.5 mg/kg doses every 5–15 min may be given; 4–5 mg/kg IM (sedation lasting 15–30 min); repeat 2–4 mg/kg IM can be given if needed after 10–15 min. Analgesia adjunct subdissociative dose: 0.01–0.5 mg/kg in conjunction with opioid analgesia.

UNAPPROVED PEDS – Dissociative sedation: Age older than 3 mo: 1–2 mg/kg IV (produces 5–10 min dissociative state) over 1–2 min or 4–5 mg/kg IM (produces 10–20 min dissociative state). Not approved for age younger than 3 mo.

FORMS – Generic/Trade: 10, 50, 100 mg/mL.

NOTES – Recent evidence suggests ketamine is not contra-indicated in patients with head injuries. However, avoid if CAD or severe HTN. Concurrent administration of atropine no longer recommended. Consider prophylactic ondansetron to reduce vomiting and prophylactic midazolam (0.3 mg/kg) to reduce recovery reactions.

MOA – NMDA receptor antagonist which produces dissocia-tive state.

ADVERSE EFFECTS – Serious: Laryngospasm, hallucinatory emergence reactions, hypersalivation. Frequent: Nystagmus, hypertension, tachycardia, N/V, muscular hypertonicity, myoclonus.

[8]DESMOPRESSIN *(DDAVP, Stimate, Minirin, Octostim)*

▶LK ⊘ ♀B ▶? $$$$$

WARNING — Adjust fluid intake downward to decrease potential water intoxication and hyponatremia; use cautiously in those at risk.

ADULT — Diabetes insipidus: 10–40 mcg (0.1–0.4 mL) intranasally daily or divided two or three times per day or 0.05–1.2 mg PO daily or divided two to three times per day or 0.5–1 mL (2–4 mcg) SC/IV daily in 2 divided doses. Hemophilia A/von Willebrand's disease: 0.3 mcg/kg IV over 15–30 mins; 300 mcg intranasally if wt 50 kg or more (1 spray in each nostril), 150 mcg intransally if wt less than 50 kg (single spray in 1 nostril). Primary nocturnal enuresis: 0.2–0.6 mg PO at bedtime.

PEDS — Diabetes insipidus: 3 mo to 12 yo: 5–30 mcg (0.05 to 0.3 mL) intranasally once or twice daily or 0.05 mg PO daily. Hemophilia A/von Willebrand's disease: (age 3 mo or older for IV, age 11 mo to 12 yo for nasal spray) 0.3 mcg/kg IV over 15–30 mins; 300 mcg intranasally if wt 50 kg or more (1 spray in each nostril), 150 mcg intransally if wt less than 50 kg (single spray in 1 nostril). Primary nocturnal enuresis: age 6 yo or older: 0.2–0.6 mg PO at bedtime.

UNAPPROVED ADULT — Uremic bleeding: 0.3 mcg/kg IV single dose or q12h (onset 1–2 h; duration 6–8 h after single dose). Intranasal is 20 mcg/day (onset 24–72 h; duration 12 days during 14-day course).

UNAPPROVED PEDS — Hemophilia A and type 1 von Willebrand's disease: 2–4 mcg/kg intranasally or 0.2–0.4 mcg/kg IV over 15–30 min.

FORMS — Trade only: Stimate nasal spray 150 mcg/0.1 mL (1 spray), 2.5 mL bottle (25 sprays). Generic/Trade (DDVAP nasal spray) 10 mcg/0.1 mL (1 spray), 5 mL bottle (50 sprays). Note difference in concentration of nasal soln. Rhinal tube: 2.5 mL bottle with 2 flexible plastic tube applicators with graduation marks for dosing. Tabs 0.1. 0.2 mg.

NOTES – Monitor serum sodium and for signs/symptoms of hyponatremia including headache, wt gain, altered mental status, muscle weakness/cramps, seizure, coma, or respiratory arrest. Restrict fluid intake 1 h before to 8 h after PO administration. Hold PO treatment for enuresis during acute illnesses that may cause fluid/electrolyte imbalances. Start at lowest dose with diabetes insipidus. IV/SC doses are approximately 1/10 the intranasal dose. Anaphylaxis reported with both IV and intranasal forms. Do not give if type IIB von Willebrand's disease. Changes in nasal mucosa may impair absorption of nasal spray. Refrigerate nasal spray; stable for 3 weeks at room temperature. 10 mcg = 40 units desmopressin.

MOA – Synthetic vasopressin analogue with a rapid onset that promotes water resorption (anti-diuretic effect). Increases factor VIII and von Willebrand's factor activity.

ADVERSE EFFECTS – Serious: Anaphylaxis, seizures (hyponatremia-associated), hyponatremia, fluid overload, chest pain, thrombotic events (rare). Frequent: Abdominal pain, flushing, headache, nasal congestion, nausea, rhinitis, agitation, balanitis, chills, increased blood pressure, sore throat, local irritation, epistaxis.

[9]TAMSULOSIN (Flomax)

▶LK ♀B ▶– $

ADULT – BPH: 0.4 mg PO daily 30 min after the same meal each day. If an adequate response is not seen after 2–4 weeks, may increase dose to 0.8 mg PO daily. If therapy is interrupted for several days, restart at the 0.4 mg dose.

PEDS – Not approved in children.

UNAPPROVED ADULT – Promotes spontaneous passage of ureteral calculi: 0.4 mg PO daily usually combined with an NSAID, antiemetic, and opioid of choice.

FORMS – Generic/Trade: Caps 0.4 mg.

NOTES – Dizziness, headache, abnormal ejaculation. Alpha-blockers are generally considered to be first-line treatment in men with more than minimal obstructive urinary symptoms. Caution in serious sulfa allergy: Rare allergic reactions reported. Intraoperative floppy iris syndrome with cataract surgery reported. Caution with strong inhibitors of CYP450 2D6 (fluoxetine) or 3A4 (ketoconazole).

MOA – Selective alpha-1 receptor antagonist that increases urinary flow rate.

ADVERSE EFFECTS – Serious: Arrhythmia, orthostatic hypotension, chest pain. Frequent: Dizziness, headache, fatigue, somnolence, edema, dyspepsia, dry mouth, nausea, palpitations, blurred vision, abnormal ejaculation.

---

[10]**MORPHINE *(MS Contin, Kadian, Avinza, Roxanol, Oramorph SR, MSIR, DepoDur, Statex, M.O.S. Doloral, M-Eslon)***

▶LK ⊗ ♀C ▶+ ©Il Varies by therapy ■

WARNING – Multiple strengths; see FORMS and write specific product on Rx. Drinking alcohol while taking Avinza may result in a rapid release of a potentially fatal dose of morphine.

ADULT – Moderate to severe pain: 10–30 mg PO q4h (immediate-release tabs, or oral soln). Controlled-release

(MS Contin, Oramorph SR): 30 mg PO q8–12h. (Kadian): 20 mg PO q12–24h. Extended-release caps (Avinza): 30 mg PO daily. 10 mg q4h IM/SC. 2.5–15 mg/70 kg IV over 4–5 min. 10–20 mg PR q4h. Pain with major surgery (DepoDur): 10–15 mg once epidurally at the lumbar level prior to surgery (max dose 20 mg), or 10 mg epidurally after clamping of the umbilical cord with cesarean section.

PEDS – Moderate to severe pain: 0.1–0.2 mg/kg up to 15 mg IM/SC/IV q2–4h.

UNAPPROVED PEDS – Moderate to severe pain: 0.2–0.5 mg/ kg/dose PO (immediate-release) q4–6h. 0.3–0.6 mg/kg/dose PO (controlled-release) q12h.

FORMS – Generic only: Tabs, immediate-release 15, 30 mg ($). Oral soln 10 mg/5 mL, 20 mg/5 mL, 20 mg/mL (concentrate). Rectal supps 5, 10, 20, 30 mg. Generic/Trade: Controlled-release tabs (MS Contin) 15, 30, 60, 100, 200 mg ($$$$). Controlled-release caps (Kadian) 10, 20, 30, 50, 60, 80, 100 mg ($$$$$). Extended-release caps (Avinza) 30, 45, 60, 75, 90, 120 mg. Trade only: Controlled-release caps (Kadian) 40, 200 mg.

NOTES – Titrate dose as high as necessary to relieve cancer or nonmalignant pain where chronic opioids are necessary. The active metabolites may accumulate in hepatic/renal insufficiency and the elderly leading to increased analgesic and sedative effects. Do not break, chew, or crush MS Contin or Oramorph SR. Kadian and Avinza caps may be opened and sprinkled in applesauce for easier administration; however, the pellets should not be crushed or chewed. Doses more than 1600 mg/day of Avinza contain a potentially nephrotoxic quantity of fumaric acid. Do not mix DepoDur with other medications; do not administer any other medications into epidural space for at least 48 h. Severe opiate overdose with respiratory depression has occurred with intrathecal leakage of DepoDur.

MOA – Opioid agonist analgesic.

ADVERSE EFFECTS – Serious: Respiratory depression/arrest. Frequent: N/V, constipation, sedation, hypotension.

---

[11]FENTANYL *(IONSYS, Duragesic, Actiq, Fentora, Sublimaze, Abstral, Subsys, Lazanda, Onsolis)*

▶L ⊗ ♀C ▶+ ©II Varies by therapy ■

WARNING – Duragesic patches, Actiq, Fentora, Abstral, Subsys, and Lazanda are contraindicated in the management of acute or postop pain due to potentially life-threatening respiratory depression in opioid nontolerant patients. Instruct patients and their caregivers that even used patches/lozenges on a stick can be fatal to a child or pet. Dispose via toilet. Actiq and Fentora are not interchangeable. IONSYS: For hospital use only; remove prior to discharge. Can cause life-threatening respiratory depression.

ADULT – Duragesic patches: Chronic pain: 12–100 mcg/h patch q72h. Titrate dose to the needs of the patient. Some patients require q48h dosing. May wear more than 1 patch to achieve the correct analgesic effect. Actiq: Breakthrough cancer pain: 200–1600 mcg sucked over 15 min if 200 mcg ineffective for 6 units use higher strength. Goal is 4 lozenges on a stick/day in conjunction with long-acting opioid. Buccal tab (Fentora) for breakthrough cancer pain: 100–800 mcg, titrated to pain relief; may repeat once after 30 min during single episode of breakthrough pain. See prescribing information for dose conversion from transmucosal lozenges. Buccal soluble film (Onsolis) for breakthrough cancer pain: 200–1200 mcg titrated to pain relief; no more than 4 doses/day separated by at least 2 h. Postop analgesia: 50–100 mcg IM; repeat in 1–2 h prn. SL tab (Abstral) for breakthrough cancer pain: 100 mcg, may repeat once after 30 min. Specialized titration. SL spray (Subsys) for breakthrough cancer pain 100 mcg, may repeat once after 30 min. Specialized titration. Nasal spray (Lazanda) for breakthrough cancer pain: 100 mcg. Specialized titration. IONSYS: Acute postop pain: Specialized dosing.

PEDS – Transdermal (Duragesic): Not approved in children younger than 2 yo or in opioid-naïve. Use adult dosing for age older than 2 yo. Children converting to a 25-mcg patch should be receiving 45 mg or more oral morphine equivalents/day. Actiq: Not approved for age younger than 16 yo. IONSYS not approved in children. Abstral, Subsys, and Lazanda: Not approved for age younger than 18.

UNAPPROVED ADULT – Analgesia/procedural sedation/labor analgesia: 50–100 mcg IV or IM q1–2h prn.

UNAPPROVED PEDS – Analgesia: 1–2 mcg/kg/dose IV/IM q30–60 min prn or continuous IV infusion 1–3 mcg/kg/h (not to exceed adult dosing). Procedural sedation: 2–3 mcg/kg/dose for age 1–3 yo; 1–2 mcg/kg/dose for age 3–12 yo, 0.5–1 mcg/kg/dose (not to exceed adult dosing) for age older than 12 yo, procedural sedation doses may be repeated q30–60 min prn.

FORMS – Generic/Trade: Transdermal patches 12, 25, 50, 75, 100 mcg/h. Actiq lozenges on a stick, berry-flavored 200, 400, 600, 800, 1200, 1600 mcg. Trade only: (Fentora) buccal tab 100, 200, 400, 600, 800 mcg, packs of 4 or 28 tabs. Trade only: (Onsolis) buccal soluble film 200, 400, 600, 800, 1200 mcg in child-resistant, protective foil, packs of 30 films. Trade only: (Abstral) SL tabs 100, 200, 300, 400, 600, 800 mcg, packs of 4 or 32 tabs. Trade only: (Subsys) SL spray 100, 200, 400, 600, 800, 1200, 1600 mcg blister packs in cartons of 10 and 30 (30 only for 1200 and 1600 mcg). Trade only: (Lazanda) nasal spray 100, 400 mcg/spray, 8 sprays/bottle.

NOTES – Do not use patches for acute pain or in opioid-naïve patients. Oral transmucosal fentanyl doses of 5 mcg/kg provide effects similar to 0.75–1.25 mcg/kg of fentanyl IM. Lozenges on a stick should be sucked, not chewed. Flush lozenge remnants (without stick) down the toilet. For transdermal systems: Apply patch to non-hairy skin. Clip (do not shave) hair if you have to apply to hairy area. Fever or external heat sources may increase fentanyl released from patch. Patch should be removed prior to MRI and reapplied after the test. Dispose of a used patch by folding with the adhesive side of the patch adhering to itself then flush it down the toilet immediately. Do not cut the patch in half. For Duragesic patches and Actiq lozenges on a stick: Titrate dose as high as necessary to relieve cancer or nonmalignant pain where chronic opioids are necessary. Do not suck, chew, or swallow buccal tab. IONSYS: Apply to intact skin on the chest or upper arm. Each dose activated by the patient is delivered over a 10-min period. Remove prior to hospital discharge. Do not allow gel to touch mucous membranes. Dispose using gloves. Keep all forms of fentanyl out of the reach of children or pets. Concomitant use with potent CYP3A4 inhibitors such as ritonavir, ketoconazole, itraconazole, clarithromycin, nelfinavir, and nefazodone may result in an increase in fentanyl plasma concentrations, which could increase or prolong adverse drug effects and may cause potentially fatal respiratory depression. Onsolis is available only through the FOCUS Program and requires prescriber, pharmacy, and patient enrollment. Used films should be discarded into toilet. Abstral, Subsys, and Lazanda: Outpatients, prescribers, pharmacies, and distributors must be enrolled in TIRF REMS Access program before patient may receive medication.

MOA – Opioid agonist analgesic.

ADVERSE EFFECTS – Serious: Respiratory depression/arrest, chest wall rigidity. Frequent: N/V, constipation, sedation, skin irritation, dental decay with Actiq.

[12] HYDROMORPHONE (Dilaudid, Exalgo, Hydromorph Contin)

▶L ⊗ ♀C ▶? ©II $$

ADULT – Moderate to severe pain: 2–4 mg PO q4–6h. Initial dose (opioid-naïve): 0.5–2 mg SC/IM or slow IV q4–6h prn. 3 mg PR q6–8h. Controlled-release tabs: 8–64 mg daily.

PEDS – Not approved in children.

UNAPPROVED PEDS – Pain age 12 yo or younger: 0.03–0.08 mg/kg PO q4–6h prn. 0.015 mg/kg/dose IV q4–6h prn, use adult dose for older than 12 yo.

FORMS – Generic/Trade: Tabs 2, 4, 8 mg (8 mg trade scored). Oral soln 5 mg/5 mL. Controlled-release tabs (Exalgo): 8, 12, 16, 32 mg.

NOTES – In opioid-naïve patients, consider an initial dose of 0.5 mg or less IM/SC/IV. SC/IM/IV doses after initial dose should be individualized. May be given by slow IV injection over 2–5 min. Titrate dose as high as necessary to relieve cancer or nonmalignant pain where chronic opioids are necessary.

1.5 mg IV = 7.5 mg PO. Exalgo intended for opioid-tolerant patients only.

MOA – Opioid agonist analgesic.

ADVERSE EFFECTS – Serious: Respiratory depression/arrest. Frequent: N/V, constipation, sedation.

[13]NORCO *(hydrocodone + acetaminophen)*

▶L ⊗ ♀C ▶? ©II $$

WARNING – Multiple strengths; see FORMS and write specific product on Rx.

ADULT – Moderate to severe pain: 1–2 tabs PO q4–6h prn (5/325), max dose 12 tabs/day. 1 tab (7.5/325 and 10/325) PO q4–6h prn, max dose 8 and 6 tabs/day, respectively.

PEDS – Not approved in children.

FORMS – Generic/Trade: Tabs 5/325, 7.5/325, 10/325 mg hydrocodone/acetaminophen, scored. Generic only: Soln 7.5/325 mg per 15 mL.

[14]VICODIN *(hydrocodone + acetaminophen)*

▶LK ⊗ ♀C ▶? ©II $$$

WARNING – Multiple strengths; see FORMS and write specific product on Rx.

ADULT – Moderate pain: 5/300 mg (max dose 8 tabs/day) and 7.5/300 mg (max dose of 6 tabs/day): 1–2 tabs PO q4–6h prn. 10/300 mg: 1 tab PO q4–6h prn (max of 6 tabs/day).

PEDS – Not approved in children.

FORMS – Generic/Trade: Tabs Vicodin (5/300), Vicodin ES (7.5/300), Vicodin HP (10/300) mg hydrocodone/mg acetaminophen, scored.

[14]LORTAB *(hydrocodone + acetaminophen)*

▶LK ⊗ ♀C ▶— ⊙II $$

WARNING – Multiple strengths; see FORMS and write specific product on Rx.

ADULT – Moderate pain: 1–2 tabs 2.5/325 and 5/325 PO q4–6h prn, max dose 8 tabs/day. 1 tab 7.5/325 and 10/325 PO q4–6h prn, max dose 5 tabs/day.

PEDS – Not approved in children.

FORMS – Generic/Trade: Lortab 5/325 (scored), Lortab 7.5/325 (trade scored), Lortab 10/325 mg hydrocodone/mg acetaminophen. Generic only: Tabs 2.5/325 mg.

MOA – Serious: Respiratory depression/arrest, hepatotoxicity. Frequent: N/V, constipation, sedation.

[14]LORCET *(hydrocodone + acetaminophen)*

▶LK ⊗ ♀C ▶— ⊙II $$

WARNING – Multiple strengths; see FORMS and write specific product on Rx.

ADULT – Moderate pain: 1–2 caps (5/325) PO q4–6h prn, max dose 8 caps/day. 1 tab PO q4–6h prn (7.5/325 and 10/325), max dose 6 tabs/day.

PEDS – Not approved in children.

FORMS – Generic/Trade: Tabs, 5/325, 7.5/325,10/325 mg.

[15]VICOPROFEN *(hydrocodone + ibuprofen)*

▶LK ⊗ ♀— ▶? ⊙II $$

ADULT – Moderate pain: 1 tab PO q4–6h prn, max dose 5 tabs/day.

PEDS – Not approved in children.

FORMS – Generic only: Tabs 2.5/200, 5/200, 7.5/200, 10/200 mg hydrocodone/ibuprofen.

NOTES – See NSAIDs: Other subclass warning.

MOA – Combination analgesic.

ADVERSE EFFECTS – Serious: Respiratory depression/arrest, hypersensitivity, GI bleeding, nephrotoxicity. Frequent: N/V, constipation, dyspepsia, sedation.

[16] PERCOCET *(oxycodone + acetaminophen, Percocet-Demi, Oxycocet, Endocet)*

▶L ⊗ ♀C ▶– ©II $

WARNING – Multiple strengths; see FORMS and write specific product on Rx.

ADULT – Moderate to severe pain: 1–2 tabs PO q4–6h prn (2.5/325 and 5/325 mg). 1 tab PO q4–6h prn (7.5/325 and 10/325 mg).

PEDS – Not approved in children.

FORMS – Generic/Trade: Oxycodone/acetaminophen tabs 2.5/325, 5/325, 7.5/325, 10/325 mg. Trade only: (Primlev) tabs 2.5/300, 5/300, 7.5/300, 10/300 mg. Generic only: 10/325 mg.

[16] ROXICET *(oxycodone + acetaminophen)*

▶L ⊗ ♀C ▶– ©II $

WARNING – Multiple strengths; see FORMS and write specific product on Rx.

ADULT – Moderate to severe pain: 1 tab PO q6h prn. Oral soln: 5 mL PO q6h prn.

PEDS – Not approved in children.

FORMS – Generic/Trade: Tabs 5/325 mg. Caps/caplets 5/325 mg. Soln 5/325 per 5 mL mg oxycodone/acetaminophen.

SICKLE CELL VASO-OCCLUSIVE PAINFUL CRISIS

Inpatient Analgesics (in the ED)	Outpatient Analgesics (discharge)
Non-Opioid	**Non-Opioid**
Oral Analgesics (if feasible): [1]**Acetaminophen:** 500 mg, best if combined with NSAIDs [2]**Ibuprofen:** 400 mg, or [3]**Naproxen:** 500 mg, or [4]**Diclofenac:** 50 mg, or [5]**Ketorolac:** 10 mg **Parenteral Regimen:** [5]**IV Ketorolac:** 10–15 mg IVP (analgesic ceiling dose) [6]**IV Lidocaine:** 1.5 mg/kg of 2% (preservative-free lidocaine-cardiac or pre-made bags only) over 10–15 min (max dose 200 mg) [7]**Ketamine (Subdissociative Dose, SDK) IV** • **IV:** 0.3 mg/kg over 15 min, +/– continuous IV infusion at 0.15–0.2 mg/kg/h • **SQ:** 0.3 mg/kg over 15 min, +/– continuous SQ infusion at 0.15–0.2 mg/kg/h	[2]**PO Ibuprofen:** 400 mg q8h × 3 days (max 5 days with 1200 mg/d) [1]**PO Acetaminophen:** 500 mg PO q8h × 3 days (max 1500 mg/day). Best if combined with [2]**Ibuprofen** at 400 mg q8h or [3]**Naproxen** at 500 mg q12h [3]**PO Naproxen:** 500 mg q12h × 3 days (max 5 days) [4]**PO Diclofenac:** 50 mg q8h × 3 days (max 5 days) **Physical Therapy** **Acupuncture** **Transcutaneous Electrical Nerve Stimulation**

(continues)

Inpatient Analgesics (in the ED)	Outpatient Analgesics (discharge)
Non-Opioid	**Non-Opioid**
• **Intranasal (IN):** 0.5–1 mg/kg (weight-based) q5–10 min (consider using highly concentrated solutions: Adults: 100 mg/mL Peds: 50 mg/mL. No more than 0.3–0.5 mL/per nostril) [8]**IV Magnesium:** 1 g over 30–45 min (as adjunct to [7]**Ketamine**) [9]**IV Haldol:** 2.5–5 mg IV (slow infusion over 10 min) [10]**IV Dexmedetomidine:** 0.5–1 µg/kg over 10–15 min (bolus); 0.1–0.2 µg/kg/h continuous infusion (range 0.1–1 µg/kg/h) with titration as needed	
Opioid	**Opioid**
Oral Regimen: [11]**Morphine:** Morphine Sulfate Immediate Release (MSIR): 15 mg [12]**Fentanyl:** Transbuccal 100–200 µg dissolvable tablets, repeat at 60 min if pain persists. [13]**Hydromorphone:** 2–4 mg	[11]**Morphine Sulfate Immediate Release (MSIR):** 30 mg q6–8h × 2–3 days [15]**Hydrocodone/ Acetaminophen (Norco)** 5/325 mg: 1–2 tabs q6–8h × 2–3 days

(continues)

Inpatient Analgesics (in the ED)	Outpatient Analgesics (discharge)
Opioid	**Opioid**
Parenteral Regimen: [11]**Morphine:** • **IV:** 0.05–0.1 mg/kg (weight-based), titrate q10–20 min • **IV:** 4–6 mg (fixed), titrate q10–20 min • **SQ:** 4–6 mg (fixed), re-administer as needed at q30–40 min • **IM:** 4–6 mg (fixed), re-administer as needed at q30–40 min (IM route should be avoided due to pain upon injection, muscle fibrosis, necrosis, increase in dosing requirements). **Nebulized** (via Breath Actuated Nebulizer [BAN]): Adults: 10–20 mg (fixed), repeat q15–20 min up to three doses Peds: 0.2–0.4 mg/kg (weight-based), repeat q15–20 min up to three doses. • **PCA:** **Demand dose:** 1–2 mg **Continuous basal infusion:** 0.5–2 mg/h	[16]**Hydrocodone/Acetaminophen (Vicodin, Lortab, Lorcet)** 5/300 mg: 1–2 tabs q6–8h × 2–3 days. [17]**Hydrocodone/Ibuprofen (Vicoprofen)** 5/200 mg: 1–2 tabs q6–8h × 2–3 days. [18]**Oxycodone/Acetaminophen (Percocet, Roxicet)** 5/325 mg: 1–2 tabs q6–8h × 2–3 days [13]**Hydromorphone:** 2–6 mg q6–8h × 2–3 days

(continues)

Inpatient Analgesics (in the ED)	Outpatient Analgesics (discharge)
Opioid	**Opioid**

[12]**Fentanyl:**
 	
• **IV:** 0.25–0.5 µg/kg (weight-based), titrate q10 min
 	
• **IV:** 25–50 µg (fixed), titrate q10 min
 	
  Nebulized (via BAN):
  Adults: 2–4 µg/kg (weight-based), titrate q20–30 min, up to three doses
  Peds: 2–4 µg/kg (weight-based), titrate q20–30 up to three doses.
 	
• **Intranasal (IN):** 1–2 µg/kg (weight-based), titrate q5–10 min (consider using highly concentrated solutions:
  Adults: 100 µg/mL,
  Peds: 50 µg/mL. No more than 0.3–0.5 mL/per nostril).
 	
• **Transmucosal:** 15–20 mcg/kg lollipops
 	
• **PCA:**
  Demand dose: 20–50 µg
  Continuous basal infusion: 0.05–0.1 µg/kg/h	

(continues)

Inpatient Analgesics (in the ED)	Outpatient Analgesics (discharge)
Opioid	Opioid
[13]Hydromorphone: • **IV:** 0.2–0.5 mg initial, titrate q10–15 min • **SQ:** 0.5–2 mg, titrate q30–40 min • **IM:** 0.5–2 mg, titrate q30–40 min (IM route should be avoided due to pain, muscle fibrosis, necrosis, increase in dosing requirements) • **PCA:** Demand dose: 0.2–0.4 mg Continuous basal infusion: 0.1–0.4 mg/h [14]Sufentanil: • **Intranasal (IN)** 0.5 µg/kg, titration q10 min up to three doses	

[1] **ACETAMINOPHEN** *(Tylenol, Panadol, Tempra, Ofirmev, Paracetamol, Abenol, Atasol, Pediatrix)*

▶LK ♀B ▶+ $
ADULT — Analgesic/antipyretic: 325–1000 mg PO q4–6h prn. 650 mg PR q4–6h pm. Max dose 4 g/day. OA: Extended-release: 2 caps PO q8h around the clock. Max dose 6 caps/day.

PEDS – Analgesic/antipyretic: 10–15 mg/kg q4–6h PO/PR pm. Max 5 doses/day.

UNAPPROVED ADULT – OA: 1000 mg PO four times per day.

FORMS – OTC: Tabs 325, 500, 650 mg. Chewable tabs 80 mg. Orally disintegrating tabs 80, 160 mg. Caps/gelcaps 500 mg. Extended-release caplets 650 mg. Liquid 160 mg/5 mL, 500 mg/15 mL. Supps 80, 120, 325, 650 mg.

[2] IBUPROFEN (Motrin, Advil, Nuprin, Rufen, NeoProfen, Caldolor)

▶L ⊗ ♀B (D in 3rd trimester) ▶+ ■

ADULT – RA/OA, gout: 200–800 mg PO three to four times per day. Mild to moderate pain: 400 mg PO q4–6h. 400–800 mg IV (Caldolor) q6h prn. 400 mg IV (Caldolor) q4–6h or 100–200 mg q4h prn. Primary dysmenorrhea: 400 mg PO q4h prn. Fever: 200 mg PO q4–6h prn. Migraine pain: 200–400 mg PO not to exceed 400 mg in 24 h unless directed by a physician (OTC dosing). Max dose 3.2 g/day.

PEDS – JRA: 30–50 mg/kg/day PO divided q6h. Max dose 2400 mg/24 h. 20 mg/kg/day may be adequate for milder disease. Analgesic/antipyretic, age older than 6 mo: 5–10 mg/kg PO q6–8h, prn. Max dose 40 mg/kg/day. Patent ductus arteriosus in neonates 32 weeks, gestational age or younger weighing 500–1500 g (NeoProfen): Specialized dosing.

FORMS – OTC: Caps/Liqui-Gel caps 200 mg. Tabs 100, 200 mg. Chewable tabs 100 mg. Susp (infant gtts) 50 mg/1.25 mL (with calibrated dropper), 100 mg/5 mL. Rx Generic/Trade: Tabs 400, 600, 800 mg.

NOTES – May antagonize antiplatelet effects of aspirin if given simultaneously. Take aspirin 2 h prior to ibuprofen. Administer IV (Caldolor) over at least 30 min; hydration important.

MOA – Anti-inflammatory/antipyretic, analgesic.
ADVERSE EFFECTS – Serious: Hypersensitivity, GI bleeding, nephrotoxicity. Frequent: Nausea, dyspepsia.

[3] NAPROXEN (Naprosyn, Aleve, Anaprox, EC-Naprosyn, Naprelan, Prevacid, NapraPAC)

▶L ⊘ ♀B (D in 3rd trimester) ▶+ $■

WARNING – Multiple strengths; see FORMS and write specific product on Rx.

ADULT – RA/OA, ankylosing spondylitis, pain, dysmenorrhea, acute tendinitis and bursitis, fever: 250–500 mg PO two times per day. Delayed-release: 375–500 mg PO two times per day (do not crush or chew). Controlled-release: 750–1000 mg PO daily. Acute gout: 750 mg PO once, then 250 mg PO q8h until the attack subsides. Controlled-release: 1000–1500 mg PO once, then 1000 mg PO daily until the attack subsides.

PEDS – JRA: 10–20 mg/kg/day PO divided two times per day (up to 1250 mg/24 h). Pain for age older than 2 yo: 5–7 mg/kg/dose PO q8–12h.

UNAPPROVED ADULT – Acute migraine: 750 mg PO once, then 250–500 mg PO pm. Migraine prophylaxis, menstrual migraine: 500 mg PO two times per day beginning 1 day prior to onset of menses and ending on last day of period.

FORMS – OTC Generic/Trade (Aleve): Tabs, immediate-release 200 mg. OTC Trade only (Aleve): Caps, Gelcaps, immediate-release 200 mg. Rx Generic/Trade: Tabs, immediate-release (Naprosyn) 250, 375, 500 mg. (Anaprox) 275, 550 mg. Tabs, delayed-release enteric-coated (EC-Naprosyn) 375, 500 mg. Tabs, controlled-release (Naprelan) 375, 500, 750 mg. Susp (Naprosyn) 125 mg/5 mL. Prevacid NapraPAC: 7 lansoprazole 15 mg caps packaged with 14 naproxen tabs 375 mg or 500 mg.

NOTES — All dosing is based on naproxen content: 500 mg naproxen is equivalent to 550 mg naproxen sodium.

MOA — Anti-inflammatory, analgesic.

ADVERSE EFFECTS — Serious: Hypersensitivity, GI bleeding, nephrotoxicity. Frequent: Nausea, dyspepsia.

---

⁴ DICLOFENAC *(Voltaren, Voltaren XR, Flector, Zipsor, Cambia, Zorvolex, Voltaren Rapide)*

▶L ✪ ♀B (D in 3rd trimester) ▶– $$$■

WARNING — Multiple strengths; see FORMS and write specific product on Rx.

ADULT — OA: Immediate- or delayed-release: 50 mg PO two to three times per day or 75 mg two times per day. Extended-release 100 mg PO daily. Gel: Apply 4 g to knees or 2 g to hands four times per day using enclosed dosing card. RA: Immediate- or delayed-release 50 mg PO three to four times per day or 75 mg two times per day. Extended-release 100 mg PO one to two times per day. Ankylosing spondylitis: Immediate- or delayed-release 25 mg PO four times per day and at bedtime. Analgesia and primary dysmenorrhea: Immediate- or delayed-release 50 mg PO three times per day. Acute pain in strains, sprains, or contusions: Apply 1 patch to painful area two times per day. Acute migraine with or without aura: 50 mg single dose (Cambia), mix packet with 30–60 mL water.

PEDS — Not approved in children.

UNAPPROVED PEDS — JRA: 2–3 mg/kg/day PO.

FORMS - Generic/Trade: Tabs, extended-release (Voltaren XR) 100 mg. Topical gel (Voltaren) 1% 100 g tube. Generic only: Tabs, immediate-release: 25, 50 mg. Generic only: Tabs, delayed-release: 25, 50, 75 mg. Trade only: Patch (Flector) 1.3% diclofenac epolamine. Trade only: Caps, liquid-filled (Zipsor) 25 mg. Caps (Zorvolex) 18, 35 mg. Trade only: Powder for oral soln (Cambia) 50 mg.

NOTES — Check LFTs at baseline, within 4–8 weeks of initiation, then periodically. Do not apply patch to damaged or nonintact skin. Wash hands and avoid eye contact when handling the patch. Do not wear patch while bathing or showering.

MOA — Anti-inflammatory, analgesic.

ADVERSE EFFECTS — Serious: Hypersensitivity, GI bleeding, hepato/nephrotoxicity. Frequent: Nausea, dyspepsia, pruritus, and dermatitis with patch and gel.

[5] KETOROLAC *(Toradol)*

▶L ⊗ ♀B (D in 3rd trimester) ▶+ $$■

WARNING — Indicated for short-term (up to 5 days) therapy only. Ketorolac is a potent NSAID and can cause serious GI and renal adverse effects. It may also increase the risk of bleeding by inhibiting platelet function. Contraindicated in patients with active peptic ulcer disease, recent GI bleeding or perforation, a history of peptic ulcer disease or GI bleeding, or advanced renal impairment.

ADULT — Moderately severe, acute pain, single-dose treatment: 30–60 mg IM or 15–30 mg IV. Multiple-dose treatment: 15–30 mg IV/IM q6h. IV/IM doses are not to exceed 60 mg/day for age 65 yo or older, wt < 50 kg, and patients with moderately elevated serum creatinine. Oral continuation therapy: 1.0 mg PO q4–6h prn, max dose 40 mg/day. Combined duration IV/IM and PO is not to exceed 5 days.

PEDS — Not approved in children.

UNAPPROVED PEDS - Pain: 0.5 mg/kg/dose IM/IV q6h (up to 30 mg q6h or 120 mg/day), give 10 mg PO q6h pm (up to 40 mg/day) for wt > 50 kg.

FORMS – Generic only: Tabs 10 mg.

MOA – Serious: Hypersensitivity, GI bleeding, nephrotoxicity. Frequent: Nausea, dyspepsia.

[6] LIDOCAINE—LOCAL ANESTHETIC *(Xylocaine)*

▶LK ♀B ▶? $

ADULT – Without epinephrine: Max dose 4.5 mg/kg not to exceed 300 mg. With epinephrine: Max dose 7 mg/kg not to exceed 500 mg. Dose for regional block varies by region.

PEDS – Same as adult.

FORMS – 0.5, 1, 1.5, 2%. With epi: 0.5, 1, 1.5, 2%.

NOTES – Onset within 2 min, duration 30–60 min (longer with epi). Amide group. Use "cardiac lidocaine" (ie, IV formulation) for Bier blocks at max dose of 3 mg/kg so that neither epinephrine nor methylparaben are injected IV.

MOA – Amide local anesthetic.

ADVERSE EFFECTS – Serious: Seizures, cardiovascular depression, bradycardia, hypersensitivity, methemoglobinemia. Frequent: None.

[7] KETAMINE *(Ketalar)*

▶L ♀C ▶? ©III $■

WARNING – Post-anesthetic emergence reactions up to 24 h later manifested as dreamlike state, vivid imagery, hallucinations, and delirium reported in about 12% of cases. Incidence reduced when (1) age less than 15 yo or greater than 65 yo,

(2) concomitant use of benzodiazepines, lower dose, or used as induction agent only (because of use of post-intubation sedation).

ADULT – Induction of anesthesia: Adult: 1–2 mg/kg IV over 1–2 min (produces 5–10 min dissociative state) or 6.5–13 mg/kg IM (produces 10–20 min dissociative state).

PEDS – Age over 16 yo: same as adult.

UNAPPROVED ADULT – Dissociative sedation: 1–2 mg/kg IV over 1–2 mm (sedation lasting 10–20 min) repeat 0.5 mg/kg doses every 5–15 min may be given; 4–5 mg/kg IM (sedation lasting 15–30 min) repeat 2–4 mg/kg IM can be given if needed after 10–15 min. Analgesia adjunct subdissociative dose: 0.01–0.5 mg/kg in conjunction with opioid analgesia.

UNAPPROVED PEDS – Dissociative sedation: Age older than 3 mo: 1–2 mg/kg IV (produces 5–10 min dissociative state) over 1–2 min or 4–5 mg/kg IM (produces 10–20 min dissociative state). Not approved for age younger than 3 mo.

FORMS – Generic/Trade: 10, 50, 100 mg/mL.

NOTES – Recent evidence suggests ketamine is not contra-indicated in patients with head injuries. However, avoid if CAD or severe HTN. Concurrent administration of atropine no longer recommended. Consider prophylactic ondansetron to reduce vomiting and prophylactic midazolam (0.3 mg/kg) to reduce recovery reactions.

MOA – NMDA receptor antagonist which produces dissociative state.

ADVERSE EFFECTS – Serious: Laryngospasm, hallucinatory emergence reactions, hypersalivation. Frequent: Nystagmus, hypertension, tachycardia, N/V, muscular hypertonicity, myoclonus.

[8] MAGNESIUM SULFATE

▶K ♀D C/D ▶+ $

ADULT — Hypomagnesemia: Mild deficiency: 1 g IM q6h for 4 doses; severe deficiency: 2 g IV over 1 h (monitor for hypotension). Hyperalimentation: Maintenance requirements not precisely known; adults generally require 8–24 mEq/day. Seizure prevention in severe preeclampsia or eclampsia: ACOG recommendations: 4–6 g IV loading dose then 1–2 g/h IV continuous infusion for at least 24 h. Or per product information: Total initial dose of 10–14 g administered via IV infusion and IM doses (4 g IV infusion with 5 g IM injections in each buttock). Initial dose is followed by 4–5 g IM into alternate buttocks q4h prn or initial dose is followed by 1–2 g/h constant IV infusion. Max: 30–40 g/24 h.

PEDS — Not approved in children.

UNAPPROVED ADULT — Preterm labor: 6 g IV over 20 min, then 1–3 g/h titrated to decrease contractions. Has been used as an adjunctive bronchodilator in very severe acute asthma (2 g IV over 10–20 min), and in chronic fatigue syndrome. Torsades de pointes: 1–2 g IV in D5W over 5–60 min.

UNAPPROVED PEDS — Hypomagnesemia: 25–50 mg/kg IV/IM q4–6h for 3–4 doses, max single dose 2 g. Hyperalimentation: Maintenance requirements not precisely known; infants require 2–10 mEq/day. Acute nephritis: 20–40 mg/kg (in 20% soln) IM prn. Adjunctive bronchodilator in very severe acute asthma: 25–100 mg/kg IV over 10–20 min.

NOTES — 1000 mg magnesium sulfate contains 8 mEq elem magnesium. Do not give faster than 1.5 mL/min (of 10% soln) except in eclampsia or seizures. Use caution in renal insufficiency, may accumulate. Monitor urine output, patellar reflex, respiratory rate, and serum magnesium level. Concomitant use with terbutaline may lead to fatal pulmonary edema. IM administration must be diluted to a 20% soln. If needed may reverse toxicity with calcium gluconate 1 g IV. Continuous use in pregnancy beyond 5–7 days may cause fetal harm.

MOA — Essential mineral needed for muscle function, organ function, potassium and calcium absorption; blocks neuromuscular transmission to prevent or control convulsions.

ADVERSE EFFECTS — Serious: Magnesium intoxication (in recipient of drug or in newborn of pregnant woman receiving Mg), cardiac depression, respiratory paralysis, hypotension, stupor, hypothermia, circulatory collapse. Frequent: Flushing, sweating, depressed reflexes.

[9] HALOPERIDOL *(Haldol)*

▶LK♀?/?/? There is evidence in humans for limb malformations when used in the first trimester. Exposure in 3rd trimester associated with withdrawal/extrpyramidal effects. ▶– $$$

ADULT — Psychotic disorders and Tourette syndrome: 0.5–5 mg PO two to three times per day. Usual effective dose is 6–20 mg/day, max dose is 100 mg/day PO or 2–5 mg IM every 1–8 h prn to max 20 mg/day IM. May use long-acting (depot) formulation when patients are stabilized on a fixed daily dose. Approximate conversion ratio: 100–200 mg IM (depot) q4 weeks is equivalent to 10 mg/day PO haloperidol.

PEDS — Psychotic disorders, age 3–12 yo: 0.05 mg to 0.15 mg/kg/day PO divided two to three times per day. Tourette syndrome or nonpsychotic disorders, age 3–12 yo: 0.05 mg to 0.075 mg/kg/day PO divided two to three times per day. Increase dose by 0.5 mg every week to max dose of 6 mg/day. Not approved for IM administration in children.

UNAPPROVED ADULT – Acute psychosis and combative behavior: 5–10 mg IV/IM, prn in 10–30 min. IV route associated with QT prolongation, torsades de pointes, and sudden death; use ECG monitoring.

UNAPPROVED PEDS – Psychosis, age 6–12 yo: 1–3 mg/dose IM (as lactate) q4–8h, max 0.15 mg/kg/day.

FORMS – Generic only: Tabs 0.5, 1, 2, 5, 10, 20 mg.

NOTES – Therapeutic range is 2–15 ng/mL.

MOA – High-potency dopamine antagonist.

ADVERSE EFFECTS – Serious: Seizures, neuroleptic malignant syndrome, extrapyramidal side effects, tardive dyskinesia, QT prolongation, sudden death, jaundice, rhabdomyolysis. Frequent: Drowsiness, nausea, dry mouth, constipation, urinary retention, hypotension, headache, hyperprolactinemia.

[10] DEXMEDETOMIDINE *(Precedex)*

▶LK ♀C ▶? $$$

ADULT – ICU sedation less than 24 h: Load 1 mcg/kg over 10 min followed by infusion 0.6 mcg/kg/h (ranges from 0.2–1.0 mcg/kg/h) titrated to desired sedation endpoint. Procedural sedation: Load 1 mcg/kg over 10 min followed by infusion of 0.6 mcg/kg/h titrated up or down to clinical effect in range of 0.2–1 mcg/kg/h depending on procedure and patient (0.7 mcg/kg/h for fiberoptic intubation). Reduce dose in impaired hepatic function and geriatric patients.

PEDS – Not recommended age younger than 18 yo.

NOTES – Alpha-2–adrenergic agonist with sedative properties. Beware of bradycardia and hypotension. Avoid in advanced heart block.

MOA – Alpha-2 adrenergic agonist with sedative properties.

ADVERSE EFFECTS – Serious: Bradycardia, heart block, hypotension. Frequent: Sedation.

¹¹ MORPHINE *(MS Contin, Kadian, Avinza, Roxanol, Oramorph SR, MSIR, DepoDur, Statex, M.O.S. Doloral, M-Eslon)*

▶L ♀C ▷? ©III $■

WARNING – Multiple strengths; see FORMS and write specific product on Rx. Drinking alcohol while taking Avinza may result in a rapid release of a potentially fatal dose of morphine.

ADULT – Moderate to severe pain: 10–30 mg PO q4h (immediate-release tabs, or oral soln). Controlled-release (MS Contin, Oramorph SR): 30 mg PO q8–12h. (Kadian): 20 mg PO q12–24h. Extended-release caps (Avinza): 30 mg PO daily. 10 mg q4h IM/SC. 2.5–15 mg/70 kg IV over 4–5 min. 10–20 mg PR q4h. Pain with major surgery (DepoDur): 10–15 mg once epidurally at the lumbar level prior to surgery (max dose 20 mg), or 10 mg epidurally after clamping of the umbilical cord with cesarean section.

PEDS – Moderate to severe pain: 0.1–0.2 mg/kg up to 15 mg IM/SC/IV q2–4h.

UNAPPROVED PEDS – Moderate to severe pain: 0.2–0.5 mg/kg/dose PO (immediate-release) q4–6h. 0.3–0.6 mg/kg/dose PO (controlled-release) q12h.

FORMS – Generic only: Tabs, immediate-release 15, 30 mg ($). Oral soln 10 mg/5 mL, 20 mg/5 mL, 20 mg/mL (concentrate).

Rectal supps 5, 10, 20, 30 mg. Generic/Trade: Controlled-release tabs (MS Contin) 15, 30, 60, 100, 200 mg ($$$$). Controlled-release caps (Kadian) 10, 20, 30, 50, 60, 80, 100 mg ($$$$$). Extended-release caps (Avinza) 30, 45, 60, 75, 90, 120 mg. Trade only: Controlled-release caps (Kadian) 40, 200 mg.

NOTES – Titrate dose as high as necessary to relieve cancer or nonmalignant pain where chronic opioids are necessary. The active metabolites may accumulate in hepatic/renal insufficiency and the elderly leading to increased analgesic and sedative effects. Do not break, chew, or crush MS Contin or Oramorph SR. Kadian and Avinza caps may be opened and sprinkled in applesauce for easier administration; however, the pellets should not be crushed or chewed. Doses more than 1600 mg/day of Avinza contain a potentially nephrotoxic quantity of fumaric acid. Do not mix DepoDur with other medications; do not administer any other medications into epidural space for at least 48 h. Severe opiate overdose with respiratory depression has occurred with intrathecal leakage of DepoDur.

MOA – Opioid agonist analgesic.

ADVERSE EFFECTS – Serious: Respiratory depression/arrest. Frequent: N/V, constipation, sedation, hypotension.

---

[12] **FENTANYL** *(IONSYS, Duragesic, Actiq, Fentora, Sublimaze, Abstral, Subsys, Lazanda, Onsolis)*

▶L ♀C ▶? ©III $■

WARNING – Duragesic patches, Actiq, Fentora, Abstral, Subsys, and Lazanda are contraindicated in the management of acute or postop pain due to potentially life-threatening respiratory depression in opioid nontolerant patients. Instruct patients and their caregivers that even used patches/lozenges on a stick can be fatal to a child or pet. Dispose via toilet. Actiq and Fentora are not interchangeable. IONSYS: For hospital use only; remove prior to discharge. Can cause life-threatening respiratory depression.

ADULT – Duragesic patches: Chronic pain: 12–100 mcg/h patch q72h. Titrate dose to the needs of the patient. Some patients require q48h dosing. May wear more than 1 patch to achieve the correct analgesic effect. Actiq: Breakthrough cancer pain: 200–1600 mcg sucked over 15 min if 200 mcg ineffective for 6 units use higher strength. Goal is 4 lozenges on a stick/day in conjunction with long-acting opioid. Buccal tab (Fentora) for breakthrough cancer pain: 100–800 mcg, titrated to pain relief; may repeat once after 30 min during single episode of breakthrough pain. See prescribing information for dose conversion from transmucosal lozenges. Buccal soluble film (Onsolis) for breakthrough cancer pain: 200–1200 mcg titrated to pain relief; no more than 4 doses/day separated by at least 2 h. Postop analgesia: 50–100 mcg IM; repeat in 1–2 h prn. SL tab (Abstral) for breakthrough cancer pain: 100 mcg, may repeat once after 30 minutes. Specialized titration. SL spray (Subsys) for breakthrough cancer pain 100 mcg, may repeat once after 30 minutes. Specialized titration. Nasal spray (Lazanda) for breakthrough cancer pain: 100 mcg. Specialized titration. IONSYS: Acute postop pain: Specialized dosing.

PEDS – Transdermal (Duragesic): Not approved in children younger than 2 yo or in opioid-naïve. Use adult dosing for age older than 2 yo. Children converting to a 25-mcg patch should be receiving 45 mg or more oral morphine equivalents/day. Actiq: Not approved for age younger than 16 yo. IONSYS not approved in children. Abstral, Subsys, and Lazanda: Not approved for age younger than 18.

UNAPPROVED ADULT — Analgesia/procedural sedation/labor analgesia: 50–100 mcg IV or IM q1–2h prn.

UNAPPROVED PEDS — Analgesia: 1–2 mcg/kg/dose IV/IM q30–60 min prn or continuous IV infusion 1–3 mcg/kg/h (not to exceed adult dosing). Procedural sedation: 2–3 mcg/kg/dose for age 1–3 yo; 1–2 mcg/kg/dose for age 3–12 yo, 0.5–1 mcg/kg/dose (not to exceed adult dosing) for age older than 12 yo, procedural sedation doses may be repeated q30–60 min prn.

FORMS — Generic/Trade: Transdermal patches 12, 25, 50, 75, 100 mcg/h. Actiq lozenges on a stick, berry-flavored 200, 400, 600, 800, 1200, 1600 mcg. Trade only: (Fentora) buccal tab 100, 200, 400, 600, 800 mcg, packs of 4 or 28 tabs. Trade only: (Onsolis) buccal soluble film 200, 400, 600, 800, 1200 mcg in child-resistant, protective foil, packs of 30 films. Trade only: (Abstral) SL tabs 100, 200, 300, 400, 600, 800 mcg, packs of 4 or 32 tabs. Trade only: (Subsys) SL spray 100, 200, 400, 600, 800, 1200, 1600 mcg blister packs in cartons of 10 and 30 (30 only for 1200 and 1600 mcg). Trade only: (Lazanda) nasal spray 100, 400 mcg/spray, 8 sprays/bottle.

NOTES — Do not use patches for acute pain or in opioid-naïve patients. Oral transmucosal fentanyl doses of 5 mcg/kg provide effects similar to 0.75–1.25 mcg/kg of fentanyl IM. Lozenges on a stick should be sucked, not chewed. Flush lozenge remnants (without stick) down the toilet. For transdermal systems: Apply patch to non-hairy skin. Clip (do not shave) hair if you have to apply to hairy area. Fever or external heat sources may increase fentanyl released from patch. Patch should be removed prior to MRI and reapplied after the test. Dispose of a used patch by folding with the adhesive side of the patch adhering to itself then flush it down the toilet immediately. Do not cut the patch in half. For Duragesic patches and Actiq lozenges on a stick: Titrate dose as high as necessary to relieve cancer or nonmalignant pain where chronic opioids are necessary. Do not suck, chew, or swallow buccal tab. IONSYS: Apply to intact skin on the chest or upper arm. Each dose activated by the patient is delivered over a 10-min period. Remove prior to hospital discharge. Do not allow gel to touch mucous membranes. Dispose using gloves. Keep all forms of fentanyl out of the reach of children or pets. Concomitant use with potent CYP3A4 inhibitors such as ritonavir ketoconazole, itraconazole, clarithromycin, nelfinavir, and nefazodone may result in an increase in fentanyl plasma concentrations, which could increase or prolong adverse drug effects and may cause potentially fatal respiratory depression. Onsolis is available only through the FOCUS Program and requires prescriber, pharmacy, and patient enrollment. Used films should be discarded into toilet. Abstral, Subsys, and Lazanda: Outpatients, prescribers, pharmacies, and distributors must be enrolled in TIRF REMS Access program before patient may receive medication.

MOA – Opioid agonist analgesic.

ADVERSE EFFECTS – Serious: Respiratory depression/arrest, chest wall rigidity. Frequent: N/V, constipation, sedation, skin irritation, dental decay with Actiq.

¹³ HYDROMORPHONE *(Dilaudid, Exalgo, Hydromorph Contin)*

▶L ⊗ ♀C ▶? ©II $$

ADULT — Moderate to severe pain: 2–4 mg PO q4–6h. Initial dose (opioid-naïve): 0.5–2 mg SC/IM or slow IV q4–6h prn. 3 mg PR q6–8h. Controlled-release tabs: 8–64 mg daily.

PEDS — Not approved in children.

UNAPPROVED PEDS — Pain age 12 yo or younger: 0.03–0.08 mg/kg PO q4–6h prn. 0.015 mg/kg/dose IV q4–6h prn, use adult dose for older than 12 yo.

FORMS — Generic/Trade: Tabs 2, 4, 8 mg (8 mg trade scored). Oral soln 5 mg/5 mL. Controlled-release tabs (Exalgo): 8, 12, 16, 32 mg.

NOTES — In opioid-naïve patients, consider an initial dose of 0.5 mg or less IM/SC/IV. SC/IM/IV doses after initial dose should be individualized. May be given by slow IV injection over 2–5 min. Titrate dose as high as necessary to relieve cancer or nonmalignant pain where chronic opioids are necessary. 1.5 mg IV = 7.5 mg PO. Exalgo intended for opioid-tolerant patients only.

MOA — Opioid agonist analgesic.

ADVERSE EFFECTS — Serious: Respiratory depression/arrest. Frequent: N/V, constipation, sedation.

¹⁴ SUFENTANIL *(Sufenta)*

▶L ♀C ▶? ©II $$

ADULT — General anesthesia: Induction: 8–30 mcg/kg IV; maintenance 0.5–10 mcg/kg IV. Conscious sedation: Loading dose: 0.1–0.5 mcg/kg; maintenance infusion 0.005–0.01 mcg/kg/min.

PEDS – General anesthesia: Induction: 8–30 mcg/kg IV; maintenance 0.5–10 mcg/kg 1V. Conscious sedation: Loading dose: 0.1–0.5 mcg/kg; maintenance infusion 0.005–0.01 mcg/kg/min.

MOA – Serious: Respiratory depression, hypotension, bradycardia, chest wall rigidity, opiate dependence, hypersensitivity. Frequent: Sedation, N/V.

[15] NORCO *(hydrocodone + acetaminophen)*

▶L ⊗ ♀C ▶? ©II $$

WARNING – Multiple strengths; see FORMS and write specific product on Rx.

ADULT – Moderate to severe pain: 1–2 tabs PO q4–6h prn (5/325), max dose 12 tabs/day. 1 tab (7.5/325 and 10/325) PO q4–6h prn, max dose 8 and 6 tabs/day, respectively.

PEDS – Not approved in children.

FORMS – Generic/Trade: Tabs 5/325, 7.5/325, 10/325 mg hydrocodone/acetaminophen, scored. Generic only: Soln 7.5/325 mg per 15 mL.

[16] VICODIN *(hydrocodone + acetaminophen)*

▶LK ⊗ ♀C ▶? ©II $$$

WARNING – Multiple strengths; see FORMS and write specific product on Rx.

ADULT – Moderate pain: 5/300 mg (max dose 8 tabs/day) and 7.5/300 mg (max dose of 6 tabs/day): 1–2 tabs PO q4–6h prn. 10/300 mg: 1 tab PO q4–6h prn (max of 6 tabs/day).

PEDS – Not approved in children.

FORMS – Generic/Trade: Tabs Vicodin (5/300), Vicodin ES (7.5/300), Vicodin HP (10/300) mg hydrocodone/mg acetaminophen, scored.

[16] LORTAB *(hydrocodone + acetaminophen)*

▶LK ⊗ ♀C ▶– ©II $$

WARNING – Multiple strengths; see FORMS and write specific product on Rx.

ADULT – Moderate pain: 1–2 tabs 2.5/325 and 5/325 PO q4–6h prn, max dose 8 tabs/day. 1 tab 7.5/325 and 10/325 PO q4–6h prn, max dose 5 tabs/day.

PEDS – Not approved in children.

FORMS – Generic/Trade: Lortab 5/325 (scored), Lortab 7.5/325 (trade scored), Lortab 10/325 mg hydrocodone/mg acetaminophen. Generic only: Tabs 2.5/325 mg.

MOA – Serious: Respiratory depression/arrest, hepatotoxicity. Frequent: N/V, constipation, sedation.

[16] LORCET *(hydrocodone + acetaminophen)*

▶LK ⊗ ♀C ▶– ©II $$

WARNING – Multiple strengths; see FORMS and write specific product on Rx.

ADULT – Moderate pain: 1–2 caps (5/325) PO q4–6h prn, max dose 8 caps/day. 1 tab PO q4–6h prn (7.5/325 and 10/325), max dose 6 tabs/day.

PEDS – Not approved in children.

FORMS – Generic/Trade: Tabs, 5/325, 7.5/325,10/325 mg.

[17] VICOPROFEN *(hydrocodone + ibuprofen)*

▶LK ⊗ ♀–▶? ©II $$

ADULT – Moderate pain: 1 tab PO q4–6h prn, max dose 5 tabs/day.

PEDS – Not approved in children.

FORMS – Generic only: Tabs 2.5/200, 5/200, 7.5/200, 10/200 mg hydrocodone/ibuprofen.

NOTES – See NSAIDs: Other subclass warning.

MOA – Combination analgesic.

ADVERSE EFFECTS – Serious: Respiratory depression/arrest, hypersensitivity, GI bleeding, nephrotoxicity. Frequent: N/V, constipation, dyspepsia, sedation.

[18] PERCOCET *(oxycodone + acetaminophen, Percocet-Demi, Oxycocet, Endocet)*

▶L ✪ ♀C ▶– ©II $

WARNING – Multiple strengths; see FORMS and write specific product on Rx.

ADULT – Moderate to severe pain: 1–2 tabs PO q4–6h prn (2.5/325 and 5/325 mg). 1 tab PO q4–6h prn (7.5/325 and 10/325 mg).

PEDS – Not approved in children.

FORMS – Generic/Trade: Oxycodone/acetaminophen tabs 2.5/325, 5/325, 7.5/325, 10/325 mg. Trade only: (Prim lev) tabs 2.5/300, 5/300, 7.5/300, 10/300 mg. Generic only: 10/325 mg.

[18] ROXICET *(oxycodone + acetaminophen)*

▶L ✪ ♀C ▶– ©II $

WARNING – Multiple strengths; see FORMS and write specific product on Rx.

ADULT – Moderate to severe pain: 1 tab PO q6h prn. Oral soln: 5 mL PO q6h prn.

PEDS – Not approved in children.

FORMS – Generic/Trade: Tabs 5/325 mg. Caps/caplets 5/325 mg. Soln 5/325 per 5 mL mg oxycodone/acetaminophen.

INDEX